YET HERE
I AM

One Woman's Story of Life After Death

DEBORAH BINNER

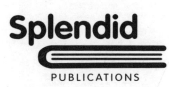

Splendid
PUBLICATIONS

YET HERE I AM

One Woman's Story of Life After Death

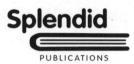

Splendid

PUBLICATIONS

Unit 7,
Twin Bridges Business Park
South Croydon
Surrey CR2 6PL

www.splendidpublications.co.uk

British Library Cataloguing in Publication Data is available from The British Library.

ISBN 978-1-909109-77-3

Commissioning Editor: Shoba Vazirani

Designed by Swerve Creative Design & Marketing
www.swerve-creative.co.uk

Printed and bound by CPI UK

**For Hannah, Roman and Nahla. And Sarah.
With all my love. Always.
In memory of Simon and Chloë. I miss you.**

———————————————

*'The only good to come from any tragedy are the lessons that can
be learnt by its survivors and their capacity to use that dreadful
experience to teach the rest of us something meaningful. In Debbie
Binner we find our heroine and our teacher. Whether loss is in
your personal vocabulary or not, this book is autobiography at
its best. If you are searching for silver linings in your clouds, then
let Debbie's journey touch you as it has me and guide you toward
meaning amongst the chaos of losing someone precious. It has been
my privilege to know this extraordinary woman. She is not only a
survivor and now, with this book, a life guide for the bereaved but
also a formidable campaigner on behalf of so many in need.
I commend her and this testament to love and living.'*
– Simon Davies, Executive Director
Teen Cancer America
www.teencanceramerica.org

———————————————

*'This is essential reading for anyone who believes that we must find
a better way to meet the needs of patients with rare diseases and will
offer comfort and guidance for anyone forced to embark on a similar
journey of grief.'*
Andy Hall, Emeritus Professor,
Newcastle University

*'What will survive of us is love. So says Philip Larkin. Debbie
Binner's wonderful story explains what this really means.'*
Maurice Saatchi

———————————————

CONTENTS

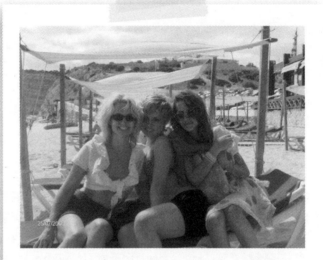

*Me, Hannah and Chloë on a wonderful
sunshine holiday. Happy times...*

PROLOGUE

'Stop worrying - nobody gets out of this world alive.'
- Clive James

FRAGMENTS OF MY LIFE

IT was a gentle breezy spring day. I was in Copenhagen with two of my closest friends. There was an unsteady contentment creeping into my life; it was a new feeling. It felt very fragile but it was nice. Gosh, Copenhagen is beautiful! We were climbing together up the stairs of the Vor Frue Kirke (Church of Our Lady) the city's main cathedral. I glanced at my friend Sian's lovely face; she was smiling.

Ah, dear Sian and her husband Mike. The kind of friends everybody needs. The people who have walked alongside me, never looking away, as the events of my tumultuous life have unfolded. They've supported me every inch of the way through two catastrophic losses. They have been outstanding friends and I am unashamed to say I love them as dearly as if they were my own family.

It was the third year that I had escaped to 'somewhere beautiful' on February 28th. A dreadful day indeed. The anniversary of the death of my precious daughter Chloë. Somehow, being outside of the UK helped. That veil of happiness that coats one on holiday is hugely helpful in times of the most terrible grief that a human can bear: the loss of a child. The beauty and promise of a new world, a contrast to the ugliness of what my family had lived through.

"Oh God, I know you." A round British woman tapped me assertively on my shoulder. "Excuse me?" I replied, assuming mistaken identity as I knew nobody in Copenhagen. Her face literally crumpled into a mixture of shock and embarrassment and the words streamed out of her mouth before she could stop them.

"Oh no, you are that poor, tragic lady from the TV. However do you cope?"

To her credit I think she would have popped the words back in if she could. Most people don't mean to be hurtful. In all fairness I had shared part of my life with a national and then international audience through the BBC BAFTA-nominated film *How to Die: Simon's Choice*. She had clearly seen me on TV at one of the darkest times of my life and seeing me later, out of context, felt she knew who I was.

Ah yes this is another whole part of my life, the death of my husband Simon. The love of my life to that point. The man who had swept me and my two young daughters up and given us the family and the love we'd never had. The man who made me laugh so much every day, with his eccentric nonsense and ferocious love of life. The man who, just one year after our Chloë had died, was struck down by the illness that is so horrific that even battle-hardened medics can barely dare to whisper its name.

Motor Neurone Disease (MND) is an uncommon condition that affects the brain and nerves. It causes weakness that gets worse over time. It's always fatal, but some people 'live' with it for many years. There's no cure but there are treatments to help reduce the impact it has on your daily life. It's caused by a problem with cells in the brain and nerves called motor neurons. These cells gradually stop working over time. It's not known why this happens.

Well that's what the NHS says about it. Here's my take: MND is the closest to a living hell that I've ever seen. It can take down the strongest person in a matter of months. If you are especially unlucky you get the Bulbar Palsy type. This is the fast-moving version which starts around the mouth, with life expectancy between six months and three years. It creeps in; a strange, tingling feeling in the tongue, speech that makes you sound drunk. Then it gets going. Choking on almost anything, coherent speech disappears leaving the sufferer to communicate with muffled noises and grunts. You fall flat on your face with no warning. Your reactions go so that you can't even put a hand out to break your fall. You whack your head on the floor again and again and again. You cough food all over the place and your breathing becomes laboured. Your arms stop working, then your legs. You shake uncontrollably and you live with the constant fear of choking to death. Your dignity is smashed into tiny pieces.

There are some gadgets that help like a walking trolley and anti-depressants have their uses - they control what the medics call 'emotional lability' which is the need to burst out crying at inopportune moments. I'd call it sanity. Who would not want to sob with such a burden to carry?

Aside from this, I really can't think of a single positive thing to say about this hideous disease. Oh, and because it's considered 'rare' - approximately affecting one person in every 50,000 with over 5,000 people in the UK affected at any one time - the pharmaceutical industry doesn't really bother with it; not enough people to make it worth the huge investment required to develop new drugs. So, no new drugs on the horizon and very little that they can do. "I'm fucked," my dear husband said. And he was.

He'd been such a proud, dignified man. A real man. Pragmatic, fiercely intelligent and brave. But also a man our little family knew it could rely on entirely. He made us feel safe and we knew beyond any doubt that he would literally kill anybody who would hurt a hair on any of our heads. He was the kind of man I would want my daughter to marry. The kind of man I'd like my grandson to grow into. A man of stature and depth. An old-fashioned Englishman in some ways.

"The endgame of MND is not to my liking," he said with characteristic understatement. He therefore became one of 37 UK residents who each year choose an assisted death in Switzerland. Not many of these however choose to have their last months on earth filmed by a BBC film crew. But my husband was unusual in many, many ways.

It was early in his illness when he could still just about speak. He burst into the room with a huge grin on his face: "Right, I'm off to Dignitas," (the more well-known Swiss assisted dying clinic) "and they are making a film of my final few months on earth. Isn't that splendid?" He told me proudly.

"And why would you do that?" I asked. His friends and family asked too. As a former TV journalist I was horrified that he wanted to expose our life and the final part of his life to a BBC audience. 'Bleeding' all over national TV. NO! NO! NO!

But I had no choice. Simon had decided and this was the first of what was to become many times that he reminded me that it was his life and he would do what he wanted with it. He said it with a mischievous smile and I knew deep down that if I'd really objected he would have changed his mind...maybe.

He was absolutely thrilled that the BBC wanted to make a film about him. Really thrilled! First and foremost it gave my hugely outgoing, attention-seeking husband a platform to tell his story. He needed it. He needed a voice as his own was being dismantled fast with this gruesome, aggressive illness. It gave his suffering some purpose, some meaning. I still don't believe he wanted to take a stand on anything in particular - he was so refreshingly honest in believing that life was tough, shit happens and then you die. "Onto the next generation," he'd announce with some gusto. But I do think it was really important for him to leave something behind. Something that mattered. I think that film mattered and still does. It shows a snapshot of a normal family coping in extraordinary circumstances. I hope that it also shows that the binary argument of whether we should have assisted dying in the UK or not, doesn't fit. It's far more nuanced than that. It needs to be agonised over and for people to get involved with the complexities of the argument. In my humble opinion, how we die is so important to how the rest of us live on.

I have spent and continue to spend a lot of time talking and thinking about death. I talk to my little grandchildren about it often. On our way back from school we regularly walk through a church graveyard and we talk and think of the bodies buried beneath us. "Can I die and go and meet all the dead people?" our little Nahla, aged four, asks breezily. "Well not really Nahla because if you died you wouldn't come back and we'd miss you," I say.

And Roman, aged six, finding Grandad Simon's shoes: "Oh no Nanny, Grandad left his shoes behind. His feet will be cold!" We listen and consider before reassuring "I think Grandad had some other shoes on so he'll be ok."

Their little minds move on to unicorns, butterflies and analysing the insects on the pavement - a particular favourite of Roman's - but they know they can return at any point to where Grandad Simon and Aunty Chloë have gone.

***

I was the child of Irish immigrants. My mother was one of 14 and had lost five siblings before she reached adulthood. Her own father died when she was 13. My father was an orphan at 14 and was pretty brutalised by the whole experience.

They were determined to protect my brother, my sister and I from what they saw as the unacceptable darkness of life, namely death. As such, as young children we were forbidden from visiting hospitals, funerals, or watching anything too sad on the TV. Elderly aunties and uncles would just seem to disappear with no explanation. The 'D-word' was never mentioned. Even hamsters and budgies would disappear without warning. It was extraordinarily confusing and it didn't work. I had never been inside a hospital until my mother got ill. I was 17 and woefully ill-equipped for what was about to happen next. More of that later.

Thankfully we talk more now don't we? But not enough. My intention is that my daughter and grandchildren will be fully informed on this subject and understand clearly that everybody dies and that we need to hold each other tighter, love each other a little more, when the inevitable happens.

Depressing? I don't think so. Learning to talk and embrace death is so much a part of living a good, meaningful, purposeful life. It also enables us to live, full, compassionate lives and to hold a hand out to those other bereaved souls. To say we are powerless in the face of death, but that we care and will walk alongside you until the loneliness subsides and you can walk on your own two feet again.

***

Back to my lady in Copenhagen. The comment still crushed me. I didn't see myself as a victim, nor was it something I ever wanted to be. I was battered, shattered and cut to the core with loss and grief. However sad my husband's death was, most especially the particular circumstances of it, my child's death 'outshone' all others in terms of misery. She couldn't have known any of this. Maybe she had a right to comment. In any case we all laughed. She apologised and I said it was all ok. And it was. At that precise moment it was. We all kind of connected in a weird, wonderful human way.

Does anyone really get grief right? It is so easy to offend when somebody doesn't have any outer skin left. But surely the best thing is to try and break through the isolation. To say something. Anything, to try and hold another person's hand when their world is falling apart around them. To show that we are all muddled, messy human beings and we often get things wrong. We are in this wonderful, chaotic, heart-breaking world together. I can forgive everything. Except silence.

***

I, an ordinary person, had shared my extraordinary life story with the general public and had therefore become something of a public person for a while. So soon with the whirl of 24/7 news I had become yesterday's 'fish and chip paper' and just another anonymous broken soul walking the earth. At the time it was a strange experience and left me wide open to other people's views on my and my family's life choices. I hated that at times, but have never wavered in my belief that it was right to share my story, our family's story. We were a family in terrible pain facing choices that we'd never have dreamt would have been forced upon us. But we really loved each other and cared deeply. Ultimately this is what saw us through in one way or another.

As a journalist I have often distanced myself from human pain by viewing the world through clever headlines, sentence construction and word counts. You have to do this to survive. As a young reporter the dreaded 'death knocks' left me as an observer in other people's desperation. Somebody else's child had died. We told ourselves that we were there to bear witness, to allow a person to tell their story. Maybe that's true. I remember every single death; I keep them in my prayers.

I felt extraordinarily vulnerable though when it came to be my turn to be the subject of the story. At the same time my family and I were all driven by a need to share our narrative. By thinking that we were somehow connecting with others and maybe even helping others in similar situations, gave us some sense of meaning and purpose. When everything you have known and loved collapses in front of you, connecting and sharing is all that is left.

The essence of my story is really about how to cope with so much death out of the natural order of things and maybe therefore about how somebody can live when the very worst of all things actually happens. I don't think you can really consider one without the other. How does one choose to live when death has a firm grip around the lifeblood of your family?

Some families just seem prone to catastrophes. You read about them in the news every day. Mine seems to be one of those families and because of that, I think my story is a useful one.

I lost my mother when I was 20. She just died one day. Sure she was ill but as I've already revealed, my family would never speak about death. She got cancer, had an operation, got better for a while and then passed away. That's all I ever really knew. I didn't know anybody else who'd lost a parent at that point, there was no internet to find a support group and not one person ever asked me if I was alright. I wasn't. In fact not for many years. Youth seems so much about movement and the future, so I was swept up with the pace of life. But I never had time to reflect on, to understand what had happened and the terrible impact it had had on me, my studies and my quality of life.

I was a bright, curious child. Resilient and ambitious. And I think that these natural qualities got me through. Propelled me to the next stage. But in hindsight I could have been more - happier, better if I'd just got some early support, had somebody stopped and asked me, "Hey how are you feeling?" But they didn't. It was a different time and place. Your mum died and you got on with it. Simple as that.

I remember people crossing the street to avoid me, maybe it was just too difficult back then. I think things are different now, but not different enough.

I was lonely and felt isolated and it took me a long time to come to terms with the idea that my mother wasn't coming back. I had a recurring dream that she was there but hiding from me. It would take many forms. Sometimes she'd be in hospital but wouldn't take my calls. At other times she'd moved to a flat but wouldn't let me in. It was always a deliberate act. She was in control trying to avoid me.

I'd wake up in a hot sweat, gasping for breath. Then the realisation that my mother hadn't deliberately abandoned me came flooding in. I'm not sure if I was more or less sad that she was instead dead and had had absolutely no choice in the matter. I'm not sure what was worse; they felt very similar.

It was years and years later that I found some peace around my mother's death. I hope that now in the age of the internet, counselling and charities that understand the needs of young people in the midst of bereavement, that people are supported through this maze of confusing feelings. I hope it's better now for others as it was pretty bleak for me and set me up for all kinds of dysfunctional behaviours and poorer outcomes. I'm quite certain if an older adult had stepped in and taken my hand, life would have been very different for me. I think I would have made different choices, better choices.

I want to explore and examine how different kinds of deaths have affected me and just maybe encourage more of us to think about death and how we support our loved ones and the members of our community who are dealing with death and dying. Isolation and loneliness are terrible bedfellows to those of us who are bereaved. By cracking open the subject and inviting our fellow humans in, surely we might be able to able to provide a better blueprint for life for our next generation.

It would be fair to say that my losses have been deep, dark and extraordinarily varied. For a westerner that is. If I lived in a third world country they may have fitted better with the normal experience of that type of society. But compared to my peers I seem to have been dealt a bit of a dud hand. First my mother and then 20 years later when I was 40, my sister. To suicide. I won't cover my sister's death here as in the midst of all the others I don't think I can do it justice. I think that suicide is one of the worst ways anybody can possibly lose someone.

The question mark left behind is all encompassing: could we have done something to prevent it? Very, very hard.

But for me the worst of the worst was my daughter Chloë's death at age 18. Completely out of the blue, she had contracted Ewing's sarcoma, at just 15, a form of bone cancer that primarily strikes in adolescence. I have heard other parents say that it's not only that they would swap places with their child in a heartbeat, but also that there is a strange lure to be with them. The brutal fact was that death - yes even through suicide - felt like the easy, warmer choice. I wanted so much to stay with her, to stay stroking her head, taking the punches right alongside. It took me a long, long time to not want to die, to not think about dying every single day. That awful feeling did eventually let up. In the end.

***

Anyway death for me at that time was really never an option. I had another child, Hannah. And as much as my heart and soul were invested in Chloë, half were also with Hannah. And by now Hannah, barely 20 years old, had two children of her own. I remember vividly the day I looked down at my own body and saw that my half a heart was still going and that actually that was probably good enough. I could live a lifetime with half a heart, as long as my other child drew breath. I have the most enormous respect for those dear brave people who cope after the loss of an only child. How they push through that early madness of grief, God only knows. They need to invent some kind of bravery medal for those people. I know two of them and I am in constant admiration of them.

Later something else happened. And, dear reader, if you are waiting for shoots of hope here's one. At first the focus must only be on putting one foot in front of the other. Don't look up, back, forward or down. Just be exactly where you are. And just by doing this something extraordinary started to happen. I started to see again. I couldn't feel for a very long time, but could see quite early on. I started to see my little family. New wondrous life – my daughter and two little grandchildren who shared my DNA. Did that really matter? Yes to me I think it did. I had felt so blighted by bad luck that this was some kind of proof that I didn't carry some dreadful curse. How could I? Look at these little beings who I'd had a part in making.

It was quite literally my grandchildren and my daughter who saved me. I am sure that I would not have lived without them. As soon as I had latched onto a purpose my sight cleared somewhat and instead of a longing for death, I started - slowly at first - to think about life. Little by little.

*****

Life is so full of contradictions don't you think? Through all of the losses, I had gained a new clarity. I'm cautious of the cliché that death and loss are transformative. My experience is that they kind of can be, but you need to work extraordinarily hard to make them so. With every fibre, every sinew of my being, I wish I'd lived a different life. I wish that what happened hadn't happened. I wish I had my family – complete with Chloë and Simon - back around me and hadn't spent so many days coiled in a foetal position wanting the world to stop. I wish I could hold my youngest child in my arms again and make it alright and stroke the little curls on her forehead and dream of the glorious future that lay ahead - a husband, more children, a relationship between two adult women who love each other so much.

But it did all happen. And it's this journey from a sheer and utter emotional tsunami to some kind of survival that I want to share. To show that even when the worst happens there is still hope and the opportunity to start again, whenever and wherever. I guess I write primarily for myself. To make sense of something. To soothe myself.

I write for my surviving child and for my grandchildren. I want them to know that sometimes life is incredibly hard, but that some sense of happiness, peace and freedom can be achieved by riding those waves and continually searching for meaning. I want them to know that it always can be ok - but only if you want it to be.

'There is freedom waiting for you,
On the breezes of the sky,
And you ask "What if I fall?"
Oh but my darling,
What if you fly?'
– Erin Hanson

And I write for you dear reader, wherever you are. I guess we pick up books like this to find some hidden secret to surviving. I know I read books for this reason and found huge comfort in the fact that others had got through equally appalling life events. I love the intimacy I find with an author. My greatest comfort has always come from literature and I include at the back of this book some of the writers who have held me with their words while I fell into tiny fragments of a human being. I haven't got any secrets I'm afraid, no magic recipes to conquer grief. All I can do is tell you what happened to me and that I somehow managed to muddle through and yes that now I have good days too.

I am such a different person now. Beaten and scarred yes, but still here. And just maybe I'm a better, kinder, more loving person in spite of it. Maybe because of it.

I listened the other day to a talk by one of my now favourite authors the lovely, ethereal Marilynne Robinson (also one of Obama's favourite writers so I'm in excellent company). Read *Gilead* if you haven't. It's life changing. If I could bottle the words and the sentiments I could live happily again. Truly extraordinary. She was wonderful to listen to. Kind but bold; strong but gentle. She's a good woman, but she doesn't suffer fools. My kind of woman.

I had been grappling with a common problem for anybody who writes. Especially one who writes personally or shares their story. I had made a clear, thought-out decision to be vulnerable, to lay-open the inner workings of my mind and soul. I don't believe anybody can write anything worth reading without exposing their deepest thoughts and fragilities. I sobbed over these pages as they capture the pain and loss. I have bashed through paragraphs of my daughter's final days and lain in emotional agony in my bed when the nightmares flooded back in. Writing hurts. And so it should if what I'm saying is important. I'm sending a report from the frontline of pain and grief - that really matters to me. My main tools are experience and honesty and I am unequivocal that this is the only way to write.

But others who have shared my journey don't make this decision. So how to write a raw, honest account but protect those whose privacy matters to them? This is a challenge. Through Marilynne Robinson's talk I found my own answer. She spoke of the care she took not to trample over the private lives of her friends and family. It somehow gave me permission. Yes I could write my truth, but I could ensure that I too stepped gently around others. I know that some of those who are nearest and dearest to me hold privacy dear, and I hope I have respected this in my story. As such I have changed names, left things out, or side-stepped. I hope in doing so that the essence of my story stands strong and true. It's a difficult balance.

***

Central to my story is other people. Through my connections and deep binds with other human beings, some friends, some health professionals and strangers too, I was able to provide a blanket of love and comfort around my child, my husband and our little family. We were never afraid to ask people to step up and they did. Human beings really can be extraordinarily marvellous when tested. Not all I know - there are some to be avoided at all costs - the 'ambulance chasers' top the list. You know those people who get their own meaning from another's misery. I can recognise them now because I am stronger. But at the worst times in my life I regretfully let people in who were not good for me and who were not good for my family. I genuinely believe that they usually have no wish to hurt, it's just that their own wounds get in the way. Simon used to say, "Hurt people hurt people." I think he was right. I lost some precious moments because I let too many people in. I regret that.

***

I am proud of my life story and I want to share it with you. The most horrible pain and heartache have turned out to be effective teachers. Long gone are the days when I'd drop everything for a chance to advance money, career and status. I relish every second I spend with my loved ones and the group of wonderful loyal friends I have around me. I watch in awe and amazement and sometimes - only sometimes - feel like the luckiest woman alive.

I've finally chosen to live and to be a new kind of happy. It's been a rocky road for sure but I hope my story provides a little light to anybody out there struggling.

***

In my darkest moments I turned to the words of Holocaust survivor Victor E Frankl:

'Everything can be taken from a man but one thing: the last of human freedoms - to choose one's attitude in any given circumstances, to choose one's own way.'

There are so many important people in my life. None of them are perfect, I don't like perfect people. An important lesson for me, through all my heartache, is to listen, to connect, to take care. I take a lot of care of my relationships now. They are by far the most important jewels in my life.

*****

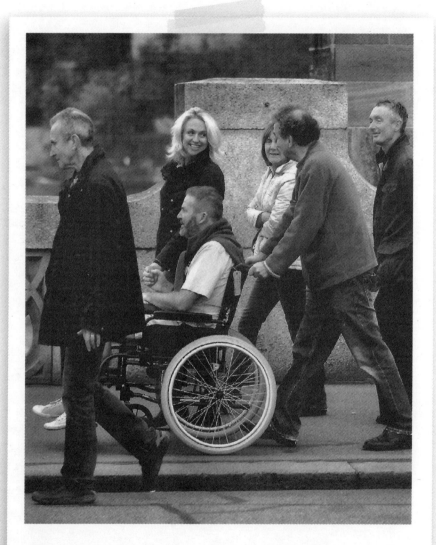

This appeared in The Sun newspaper as Simon prepared to die in Basel — he was actually delighted!

ONE

SIMON'S CHOICE

November 2nd 2013

To my dear husband Simon, on your 54th birthday,

Well we've been married 12 years now. As you always say, "It certainly hasn't been boring."

We've been through the worse thing any parents can ever go through - the loss of our daughter Chloë. It's been so sad and so difficult and at times I wasn't sure we'd make it. I'm not the person I was and I know that life has just been made so hard. But I think we're pulling through. With you, I've simply had the most fun I've ever had in my life. You make me laugh. What a gift! And you've loved my daughters like they were your own. I never expected that. Of course you are the most annoying person in the world too! When we first met I knew we'd have fun. And I would have settled for that. I had no idea of the hidden depths of loyalty, love and kindness you would show me and my loved ones. You cared for my dad when I was busy with Chloë's cancer and then you cared for us all as we put everything we had into making sure every second of Chloë's life was worthwhile. Not once did you ever complain. We need to heal together now and put some of our life back together. There is still lots of life and fun to have. And I have no doubt we'll be off on the next stage of our adventure together. You've shown me the meaning of the word love. You've restored my faith that a man can be loyal, faithful and entirely trustworthy. You are my rock and I love you with all of my heart.

Your wife
Debbie

***

IT was October 19th 2015 at 11am. We were in Basel in north western Switzerland on the River Rhine. The previous day I had walked with my husband Simon hand in hand in the sunlight across Mittlere Brucke (Middle

Bridge) the oldest bridge in the town. Can you believe I'd read the guide book and for a tiny moment got excited at the prospect of exploration.

I'd noticed momentarily a very tall, well-dressed man on the bridge. He had a camera. My journalist instincts kicked in. He looked out of place. It didn't come as a huge surprise when a picture of me, Simon's sister Liz and three of the friends who accompanied us, appeared the next day on the front of *The Sun* newspaper. 'Hand in hand,' it screamed as it told the world that we were about to end Simon's life at a Swiss suicide clinic.

Of course. I'd spent my working life as a journalist and should have realised that this was a newsworthy story. Simon had posted on his LinkedIn account the date of his death! October 19th 2015. He'd signed off as usual "Ebullient regards." He said he'd had a blast, but motor neurone disease (MND) was taking him down fast. 'Assisted dying', 'successful businessman' (this had turned into 'multi-millionaire' - if only!) and a social media announcement. Some of the news headlines leading up to Simon's death. It must have been a quiet news day to make the front page of a national newspaper.

Simon feasted his eyes on the newspaper and chuckled knowingly. By then he'd lost his power of speech and communicated with us by pen and paper. He could still just about write, although even that was simply, "Ha, look we've made it to the front page of *The Sun*." In a strange coincidence somebody we knew by association knew the photographer who had taken this picture. Much later he rather apologetically sent me a framed copy of the photo and passed on that they had only followed in as unobtrusive fashion as possible to see if they could cover the story. If only they'd known how much Simon had enjoyed the chase! Our friends and I were less impressed, but Simon found it hugely amusing. If only he'd reached this level of attention whilst he was alive. Well that would have been a thing. So no harm done really and in all truth *The Sun* helped to make a dying man very happy that day.

Basel's old town is one of the best preserved in Europe. On every corner one can find buildings dating back as far as the 15th century. The stunning cathedral is Basel's most well know trademark. The Pfalz viewing terrace behind the cathedral offers a lovely view of the city and the Rhine. The City Hall, or Rathaus building, with its eye catching red facade has beautiful frescoes to admire.

It was indeed a beautiful chocolate box type of town, with cobbled streets and a mystical air of expectation. That feeling of hope and anticipation that one gets at the start of a holiday. Ah Basel I shall not be returning in this lifetime I'm afraid. Unless of course… well, let's not go there.

But we were not there to explore, to fill our minds with the histories of another town and life. We were there for an entirely different purpose.

We had met Dr Erika Preisig earlier that summer. Her diminutive figure belied a staunch unfaltering belief in the courage of her own convictions. The result was a kind of human dynamo. She was mesmerising and had an ethereal quality to her personality that so drew me in. I think it comes from an authenticity, a belief in something so strong and for the most noble of reasons, that the person seems to rise above ordinary life. I've seen it only a couple of times before. It's a beautiful thing.

So why Erika? And why not Dignitas which after all is the most well-known assisted dying clinic?

This is a difficult question to answer as I'm afraid that some of the detail has faded as one moves away from the pain of the trauma. I wish I'd written more. Remembered the detail. It matters. I don't know why it matters, but it does. I think we chanced upon Erika as Simon was doing some research. We had at first thought Dignitas was the only option available, but then discovered that Eternal Spirit had been set up by Dr Preisig to provide an alternative. We immediately liked her approach. She had worked with Dignitas but had broken away to provide a solution that was far more aligned to working with palliative care and although she didn't say as much, maybe a more personalised approach. All of our dealings with Eternal Spirit, from start to finish, were with Erika personally. I have to say if I were ever to consider this path - and I hope never to be in this position - Erika would be top of my list. I'd give her a five out of five on my 'death experience' Trip Advisor score.

Erika was, is, a conviction doctor. Anybody could see that. She was utterly, one hundred per cent convinced that people suffered less by having an assisted death. I'm not sure I've ever met anybody quite so certain in her beliefs, yet who was entirely without any personal vanity. Others I met sometimes seemed to relish the controversy and attention that their stance gave them - on more than one occasion I wondered how much this minor celebrity status was at least one of the reasons behind their campaigning. Speculation of course.

But I remain puzzled by Erika's passion, which at times seemed to veer towards obsession. She had worked for many years as a GP in the Swiss mountains. A place where you can taste the sweetness of life in the clearness of the air. It had unnerved me that the pro-assisted dying lobby, seemed to 'sell' it as some kind of panacea to all of life's ills. A kind of flippancy around the process of dying: you're worn out; it's time to go. But Erika was different. Unswerving in her belief? Yes definitely. But, and I looked straight into the whites of her eyes, driven entirely by a desire to alleviate human suffering. Not to cause any.

Yet I still kicked against her view. I still do to a large extent - although as time goes on and my thoughts settle, less so. My head understands all the intellectual arguments and I find it hard to disagree. But my heart still says no. Should we not be kinder, more patient, more respectful of human life? Isn't how we support the dying so central to who we are as human beings?

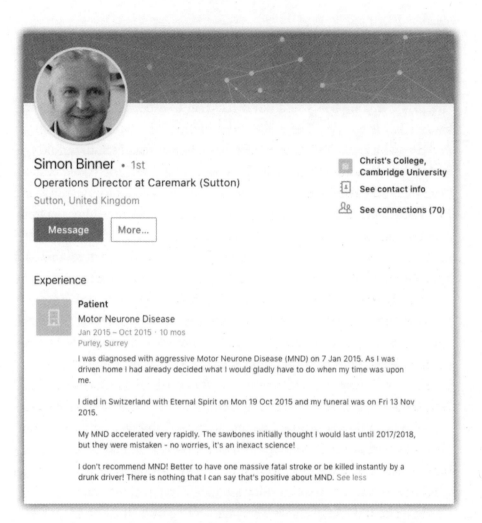

Simon's LinkedIn post bidding farewell to the world
in typical Binner fashion.

***

Some dismiss my view and put it down to a Catholic upbringing. I don't agree. It's something else and I've never done very well in capturing what I want to say. I think it's about value. The value we put on life. On love. On family. I worry deeply about how people who are ill can lose the sense of mattering to other people.

When my own Chloë was close to the end of her life she said to me, "Mum, I bet you wish you'd never had me. I've been a bit of a defect, haven't I?" Jesus! At 17 she felt like a burden. She wasn't anything of the sort and it broke my heart to hear her talk like that. Nothing could be further from the truth. I'm not sure I could have loved my daughter any more than I did. But when she was ill my love stepped into another gear. My whole raison d'être was in making her life the best it could be. I cared about nothing else. The fact she felt she was less than anybody else because she had cancer was abhorrent to me. That Simon felt his life wasn't worth living because he felt "unmanly" and "undignified" upset me too.

I've since questioned myself on this. Did caring for Chloë give me purpose? Was I really motivated by wanting to be a kind of Florence Nightingale figure? Did Simon really need protecting from somebody like me who would have been quite content to devote my every second to him as a kind of 'human pet.' Ha, those were the words that Erika used. Did I want Simon as a 'pet?' A little harsh, but I think that there is an issue here.

I genuinely do not believe I was motivated by that. As a matter of fact I was never drawn to a caring profession. I'm great in a crisis - true. And I understand that sometimes a crisis does give one purpose that ordinary life doesn't always provide. It shifts the focus from me, me, me to another person. A by-product of this is a strange feeling of well-being. I get that. I've heard some people who have lived very traumatic lives, struggle to cope when life becomes calm again. They don't know what to do with all those coping strategies. Yet, even though I accept these as valid arguments, I don't believe that a law which allows assisted dying is good for a society. I think we struggle enough with valuing people who don't fit with our norms. Over time I believe it would seep into our collective consciousness and that would adversely colour how we view people who were sick, disabled, old. It's bad enough now.

***

I've always veered towards the minority. As a child I felt so disconnected myself - normal on the outside but hiding terrible family secrets of mental illness and alcoholism. Ordinary society accepted me. I was popular. I looked right, spoke right. Sometimes I used to giggle to myself thinking, "If only they knew." Behind our beautiful manicured lawn, cut glass sherry decanters and a rose bush around the door - there was utter chaos and misery. Middle class misery. Really the same misery as anywhere else, only it seemed almost worse as it was so hidden.

I was a red-headed Irish Catholic girl, born only a decade after the infamous 'No blacks, no dogs, no Irish' signs on shop windows. My mother felt prejudice deeply and had elocution lessons to drown out her Irish lilt. Ha, she would have laughed so much to see me and my brother hastily filling in our Irish passport applications ahead of the madness of Brexit!

We outsiders seem to understand each other. Like a hidden language. I'm grateful for my background in some ways. I'm proud to say I've inherited my parents' most wonderful qualities - empathy and a consistent ability to always see the humanity and dignity in others no matter what their circumstances. My mother would have greeted the Queen in exactly the same way that she embraced the homeless, friendless, elderly Irish ladies who sat around our festive table. "I'll not see anybody be lonely at Christmas," she'd say. She had this way of making everybody feel that they mattered. I was very proud of her for that.

I also think of the elderly people - mums and dads - in my friends' lives and how important they are to their functioning, the functioning of their family, of the wider community. My own mother-in-law is 89 and she is adored so much. She remains massively important to me and the rest of her family. One of the most tender things I've ever seen is my grandson looking up at my mother-in-law with large trusting eyes. He loves spending time with her. She's important to his well-being. Caring for each other can bring out the very best in each of us. I worry that if we allowed assisted dying here it would somehow devalue these lives that might not be considered 'economically viable.' Yet nobody wants their loved ones to suffer more than necessary.

I'm extremely glad that I don't have to make this decision. I only hope that by sharing life from the frontline of assisted dying it can somehow input into a deep and thoughtful debate.

I get the suffering. I've seen it up close and personal. My husband was more afraid of living than dying. I have never seen anybody who wanted to die so much. He loved all of us and he was fundamentally a loving and kind man. His struggle was how to shake me off and leave me and our two remaining children intact. I know he hated leaving me and our daughters, but he couldn't go on. I think there were moments when he wished that we hadn't loved him so much. He would have been freer to follow his own path. Ultimately, we became a bit of an annoyance to him - in the nicest possible way.

So why did I go with him to that Swiss clinic? Why didn't I take a stand, if not for me and my family, for all the other families that could come afterwards? Me, somebody who'd fought so hard not to go. Well it went like this. One day I plucked up the courage and said, "I'm not coming with you." He looked at me half amused. "OK," he wrote. We'd had a feisty relationship before now, even through his illness, so I'd expected a fight. Believe me he was pretty good at conveying his emotions through blazing eyes and the flick of his pen. But this time he was just tender. "I want you to be ok," he wrote. "I don't want to cause you any more hurt. But I have to go. I can't do this."

I walked away, tears pooling in my eyes. He'd fight me, but always give in in the end. I'd played my last card and it hadn't worked.

***

It was two or three days later. My decision was still hanging in the air. But things were ok and what happened next seemed to come completely out of nowhere. I was in the kitchen. Other people were there. I think the dog walker was there. But their presence faded fast as my daughter Hannah screamed "NO!" All eyes to the garden. Autumn was coming, the leaves were turning. The tree swing, where my little girls had spent hours of amusement swinging high up in the glorious horse chestnut trees, was in view. A childhood swing. Happy memories of a normal family at play. Simon, who at this point could hardly shuffle let alone walk, had somehow got himself to the end of the garden - and it was a long way out there. He'd taken the swing rope and wedged it around his neck. As impossible at it seemed he'd dragged a step ladder out too. My husband, the loving family man, was about to hang himself on our children's swing. What! This was total madness.

We raced to the patio doors. They were locked. He'd locked us in. This was no cry for help. Simon was so far from being a cruel, unkind man; this was so out of character. In hindsight I feel that the utter desperation of his plight, my refusal to go with him to Switzerland and the terrible bleakness of the illness had driven him momentarily mad. He just couldn't see another way out.

It is hard to include the details of this part of our life. But I think it is critical evidence. Here was a man who was so terrified of living that he was driven to do the unthinkable.

Hannah, who'd been a brilliant young runner, sprinted around the front of the house and got to him. Us adults were trapped inside. She was the best person to go as most of all he would not have wanted to hurt the children. He looked chastised as she told him off. Ha, what a strange thing that was, my young daughter reading him the riot act.

Some tears and some hugs. They came back inside. I felt so angry with him; but so sympathetic too.

He seemed shaken and we helped him back up to bed. He started to sob gently and I held his head in my lap - like a child. I felt so terribly sad for him, for me, for us. He asked me to read him some poetry. I did and he calmed slightly. We used to love reading poetry to each other. It was part of our love story.

I wanted to shout at him: "What the hell were you doing! The children's swing! In front of Hannah!" But I couldn't. I couldn't because I was starting to really understand. This was a man who really, really wanted to die; not because he didn't love all of us, but because he was utterly terrified of having to carry on living.

I went downstairs and 'phoned our friend Simon Sandberg. I dragged him out of a work meeting. He didn't hesitate and neither did Sian or Mike. Our little troop who formed a warm blanket of love and support around us whenever it was needed. They were by Simon's bedside within the hour.

Leaving just enough time for Simon's second suicide attempt.

I'd gone down to make a cup of tea. Hannah had left the house. But something brought her back in. A sixth sense? She bolted up the stairs to our loft room and there he was again trying to jump out of a window. But he could hardly walk, move even! How ever did he find the strength? Sheer pig-headed determination and desperation of course. It was all so utterly, utterly heartbreaking. His actions certainly were speaking far louder than any words he could write.

We got him back down, back into bed, and we sat around his bedside. Shaken, distraught, exhausted.

Later that evening I took his hand. "I'll come," I whispered. "I'll arrange it now." His face crumpled into what can only be described as complete relief. I'd underestimated how important my presence, my blessing was to the whole thing. We'd always done things together.

I looked into his bright blue eyes, the eyes I'd fallen in love with, and understood - really understood - what this man wanted. There was no denying it anymore. He needed to die and on that day it became very clear to me that there were worse ways to die than to travel to an organised Swiss clinic. At least we could prepare, group around him and say a proper goodbye. An unplanned suicide really would have been the worst of all eventualities.

And I guess at the end of the day this is what love expects of all of us.

That we act entirely selflessly at times. After this day I didn't feel that I had any choice to make. I had to go. It was my duty. And in hindsight I believe I made the right decision.

That night I called Erika and explained what had happened. Her sweet, gentle voice made everything seem ok again. She made Simon promise that he wouldn't try anything else and then said she'd put off a trip so that she could personally provide my husband's assisted death.

**

I cannot think of a better person to accompany a devastated family on this particular journey than Erika. She helped my husband enormously. She listened and gave him a solution when nobody else could. If assisted dying is something on your radar I would, without question, recommend this remarkable woman. Whilst not entirely buying into her chosen path, I do appreciate she is so obviously driven by a love of humanity. And maybe if everybody I had met had been like Erika I would feel warmer to the idea of assisted dying - it's just us humans are a mixed bunch aren't we?

**

In Basel was Liz, one of Simon's two sisters and our friends Mike, Simon and Will.

My Simon and I had worked hard together to decide who should be there. It was a tortuous decision as we knew we would cause pain by leaving some people out. And probably pain by including people too. Attending an assisted death may not, as my husband joked, be somebody's idea of "a good night out."

We could not ignore the fact that anybody who accompanied us could have been arrested and faced a maximum of 14 years in jail. It was highly unlikely, but the law remains clear on this point and it was something that needed to be considered. No lawyer could reassure us that we wouldn't be arrested, even though the current trend means that the law turns a blind eye unless it suspects foul play. Meaning that in effect assisted dying is kind of legal with a few provisos - you need at least £14k to arrange it and nerves of steel. You need to step outside of the warmth and comfort of the NHS and go it alone. You can't talk about it with anybody else and there's no counselling or anything else that is going to pick you up. Dignity in Dying, the organisation that campaigns for a change in the law in the UK to allow an assisted death here, accuses the UK of 'out-sourcing' compassion. I can't argue with this.

The fine doctors at King's College Hospital, a centre of excellence for the 'treatment' of MND were as supportive as they could be within the law. Among the outstanding team there was a Dr. Rachel Burman, a palliative care specialist. She prodded and explored Simon's reasoning and this was so helpful. She stayed curious and expressed a desire to "walk alongside" as this horrible disease progressed. She was powerless in having no treatment to offer - there isn't one - but her desire to stay close and see it through to whatever ending came about was genuine, tender and made me, especially, feel less alone.

Being a MND specialist is a tough gig. Day after day of seeing people step out of the world of the well and into a parallel universe with a whole series of physical and mental tortures to be worked around or simply endured. With MND people often talk of Stephen Hawking and how worthwhile – and long - his life was. Closer to my home is a friend's father who was given a death sentence at 44 and lived, quite happily apparently, until 86. As a scientist and an academic he lived in his mind and then on his computer.

I secretly hoped that this would be Simon too. Selfishly I needed him. He was my guide and my rock. There were two points against me. Firstly Stephen Hawking and my friend's dad were serious outliers. The path of MND is usually far faster and more brutal. Secondly, with Simon it took his voice and language first when words and conversation were his very core. Nothing could have been more painful for Simon and I do believe that being unable to communicate made his life not worth living to him at least. He said he could have lived better with the physical challenges. But he was a great communicator and taking this away attacked the very heart of who he was. We heard of a rugby player whose MND had started in his legs. For him the physical restrictions were worse.

Like so many things, it all depends on who you are. A reminder that judgements about others are often useless and sometimes even offensive as they deny the person's unique personality.

"All we can do is walk alongside you. We will listen for however long it takes and we will never turn away."

Such wise words from Dr. Rachel Burman and for me a real clue how we can all help someone we love when the very worst happens.

There are some theories that MND is linked to highly active people and sports people appear to be slightly more affected than the general population. There are other views that very high energy people are more vulnerable.

But these are theories, nothing proven. Just hunches. In my bleak journey through these disease groups I've often felt how come that we can send a man to the moon, access so much at the touch of the button, but we seem to know so little really about the human body and especially about these so called 'rarer' illnesses.

***

Simon was 56 and highly active. He was a poor sleeper and drove himself hard. Simon's consultant Professor Ammar Al-Chalabi admitted that there is a sound reason why he could have tried an HIV treatment. Would it have worked? Highly unlikely. Since Chloë died I've worked tirelessly campaigning for better access for newer and kinder drugs for children and teens with cancer. Early drug development is really only about determining safety and monitoring side effects and by far the huge majority of drugs are dropped as they just don't make any difference. There are so few breakthrough drugs - in fact people still point to penicillin as being the last real blockbuster drug. There are improvements and shifts and it's true that more people live longer, better lives in a number of disease groups such as childhood leukemia, cystic fibrosis and even breast cancer.

What makes me mad is that nobody is throwing bricks through windows shouting, "What about the rare illnesses!" So what if they don't make money. Aren't we better than that as a society, as a human race?

The fact is if you are unlucky enough to get an illness like MND there is no treatment for you and never will be unless something in the system changes. Unless a new model of drug development emerges that allows the public sector or the charity sector to share some of the risk with industry. It would be good for society as it would be fairer. It's not the person's fault that they happen to get a rare illness as opposed to a common one. It is, in my experience, also really important for the person. It gives them hope. A trial drug may have just given Simon a reason to go on a bit longer and that would have been good for all of us.

And there's that purpose thing again. Simon had lost his reason for being. But he would have liked to contribute to medical science. I think sometimes we underestimate how altruistic us humans can be given the chance. Just maybe something good could have happened. A slowing down of a particular side effect perhaps. It is the absence of hope that is so very difficult to live with. I've seen doctors roll their eyes when this is mentioned as if this is way out of their pay scale.   "Well   people might want hope, but there isn't any and we can't run a system - already buckling under the strain - on peddling hope." And maybe if pushed I'd agree with this. But hope as a by-product of more, better drug development that is providing those much needed clues on the very, very long path to finding something that may work, or at least genuinely alleviate symptoms, well that's a different matter.

But Simon wasn't allowed to hope. I know only too well from the treatment of childhood cancer that a serious block to development of these new drugs is ROI – the return on investment of huge costs against the few numbers of people who will need the drug. You can see that in our current system private companies are going to get far more excited about drugs for lung or breast cancer than they are for rarer illnesses affecting so few people.

***

Back to Simon's choice. We'd been warned by doctors at King's College Hospital that anybody involved with an assisted death was likely to be adversely affected. That it was a 'complicated death' for others to deal with. For this reason we decided against allowing Simon's mother Jean to accompany us to Basel or our two daughters Hannah and Zoe (Simon's daughter from his first marriage). In hindsight I think we were right about our girls. I don't think that young people need to see something like this. I'm not entirely sure about Jean though. Simon was her child. Maybe she should have come. What I do know is that we thought everything through as thoroughly as we could at the time and we came up with the best list we could. But I know we hurt some people along the way. And for that I'm sorry.

In Basel on the evening of October 18th we ate a final meal. I'd planned carefully what I would wear. I had a really pretty red blouse that Simon loved. It was cold, I would have preferred a big snug jumper but I still wanted to dress up for my husband. Even then. One final time. He told me that I looked beautiful. He so often told me that. It was so precious. Every woman should marry a man who looks at them the way that Simon looked at me. I'd spent so many years with the wrong kind of man and it was only through meeting Simon that I understood how much more magical life is with the right life partner. He was always by my side. Always on my side. We went down to dinner with our friends, just like we had done hundreds of times before. We'd holidayed with many of these people and had eaten with them in restaurants across the world. It seemed like the most normal thing in the world. In one way.

It was only when I looked at the menu that my head started to swim. This was the very last meal I would eat with my husband. I had become used to being on standby for a choking incident. That happens a lot with MND. At first it's simply embarrassing. Then it's just plain scary. Then it becomes part of the meal. By the end I was almost blasé in readying myself for the slap on the back, pushing his head forward. If that didn't work it would be a fist under the rib cage. How strange how these things start to become normal. I also couldn't care less who was watching. That said one often sees the best of humanity in the worst of circumstances. All I saw was people trying very hard to help.

So surreal, the BBC crew was with us too. I know they always felt slightly embarrassed that they were gatecrashing a final party. I'm not sure they ever knew how important they were to Simon and me. Both of us needed people around us. Being alone with this would have been too much to bear. Isolation. Lack of connection. For me and most definitely for Simon, these would have been too hard. For others the opposite would have been true I guess. The fact that his story would be broadcast after he had gone, gave him peace. It gave him and me to some extent, purpose. Our fate was well and truly sealed. All that was left was a choice to help others by sharing our story. He was going to leave a footprint, a legacy and this was really comforting to him. I know so many people ask why ever did you open your life up like this to a public audience? I know that some will say why write a book? Go back quietly to normal life. To us we thought why ever would we not? And for me there is no normal life anymore. It was a human story about a subject that needed talking about. I remain really pleased that we made the film and I hope that writing this book helps someone somewhere feel less alone. I'm not sure I will ever watch that film again though. It's just too painful. But through the thousands of letters, emails and messages I have since received from across the world I know it has made a difference and helped people. That has given me huge comfort. It's that connection thing again.

***

Simon gobbled his dinner down. He'd have loved a steak, but that was another pleasure he'd been denied for a long while by the time we sat down for our final meal. One of the numerous challenges of MND is that chewing and swallowing become difficult early on. Food needed to be soft, or by the time we got to Switzerland it really needed to be pulverised. Although typical Simon spurned most medical devices and would have none of the liquidised stuff. He would immediately have choked on steak. He was still just able to eat softer foods and I think, although it's mainly a blur, he ate

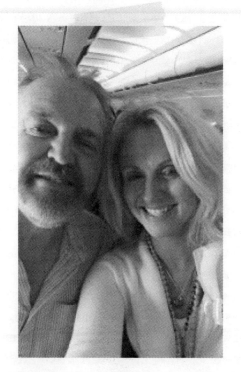

With Simon on the plane to Basel looking like excited tourists. If only the other passengers knew...

lightly cooked fish and mashed potato. Our friend Simon recalls the food as being "pretty awful." I have absolutely no idea what it was like. If I put a morsel to my mouth I can't remember. It was at that moment I was struck by the most awful dread. We were fast running out of time. My husband was slipping away. He took my hand and smiled.

We shared Simon stories around the table. I remember dear Mike talking of how much he had "belly laughed" at all the years of Simon's practical jokes and general nuttiness. Something so tender about male friendships at this stage of life. Liz, his sister, spoke with no bitterness at all of how Simon was the "most loved" young Binner. How he would steal the spotlight at every opportunity. She didn't mind. None of us minded that Simon was always the centre of attention. It's just who he was and that was just fine. I always felt that it was a fitting conclusion to the narrative of his life - larger than life doing everything on his terms. Why would I have expected the end to be any different?

Surrounded by people who loved him so dearly, he was not going to fade into old age with more indignities. Be left in an old folks' home and be grateful for the odd visit. Oh no, he'd cheated us all of that one. He was going out in a flash of glory. Surrounded by friends and family and the star of his very own TV documentary. Only somebody with the flamboyancy, flair and bloody mindedness of my Cambridge-educated husband could orchestrate their final moments like this.

And he seemed happy. Honestly really happy and at peace. I was amazed. A local Swiss GP visited as part of the process. He had one of those Christmas jumpers on with a reindeer and some snowdrops around it. It looked funny and Simon and I shot a knowing 'Ha, Swiss man out of central casting' look. I have no idea what his name was, but he sauntered in with a calm, breezy air. More like he was greeting old friends for a few drinks than signing away the last part of somebody's existence. He made sure that Simon understood what he was doing. I asked if it would hurt. It was suddenly incredibly important to me that nothing more would hurt Simon in any way. He said it wouldn't and I believed him. Everybody seemed so genuinely well motivated in this very strange final scene.

We had been warned of a 'conveyor belt' process where people are 'herded in and out one after the other' into a kind of soulless death chamber. It wasn't like that. Compared to the grisly stories of elderly people dying in busy hospital wards, or even corridors, in our own UK health system, this death was being so carefully planned. A lot more thought through.

I know, I know. I make a good case for assisted dying. But something stops me from wholeheartedly endorsing it. More than anything I think it's the slippery slope argument. It was ok for Simon. It would be ok for me. But would it be good for a society that so often turns a blind eye to people with rubbish luck? And, in my view, the after effects on the family and friends are especially complicated.

***

We ended our evening - the night before Simon died - alone in our bed. I helped him off with his clothes and combed his hair. He always liked his hair nicely presented. He couldn't speak at all by this time, just made a distressing grunting noise. I held him gently in my arms as his breathing became heavier and heavier. We said nothing. I think we'd both said everything that needed saying. There was a strange calm and peacefulness in the room. There was no going back now. This was the end of our lovely love story.

***

MONDAY 19TH OCTOBER 2015

Was I imagining it or were people in the hotel looking at us strangely. There has since been quite a lot of opposition in Basel to foreigners using their assisted dying service. Not a great tourist draw. I was a little surprised that the issue of assisted dying seems to be as controversial in Switzerland, where it has been legal since 1942 as long as 'the motives are not selfish,' as it does in the UK. It did not feel like a closed case even here. And I felt we were creeping about under the radar and that people may have been watching. May have been judging. Or was I the one judging? Never completely convinced this was the right thing to do, I was my biggest critic.

Mike came to our room and helped Simon to dress. A middle-aged man helping his middle-aged friend one last time. Mike's face was drawn but determined. He would miss him dreadfully. I think Liz turned up too. Dear brave Liz. She was there to see her big brother die. The tears were pooling in her eyes, but she didn't let on. She just joined us. We went down and met the other Simon and Will at breakfast.

The taxi arrived and here I go blank. I think Simon was sitting in the front and the boys with me and Liz in the back. It was Simon, or was it Mike, who held my hand. I'd long since stopped crying after my daughter had died and I didn't think I had any tears left. I was mistaken. My Simon glanced in the mirror and saw the big fat tears streaming down my cheeks and his face crumpled. I knew that he was so very sorry for leaving me. He'd spent the last 14 years protecting me, helping me to make sense of the world. He said he felt he was letting me down by leaving early. He knew I didn't want him to go; but he knew he couldn't stay either. I know that he died knowing that he was utterly adored by so many people. A man who always put me first had to continually, gently, explain that I had to go and live my life without him. He was an extraordinary man.

We ended up by a strange kind of shop front. We went in. It was not a shed as some had warned. It was a nice enough room with a bed and a table and chairs. I think that there were paintings on the wall and lots of CDs around. Erika was standing there in her usual little signature plaits, hair styled in such a non-threatening Heidi kind of way. Quite at odds with the reason she was there.

Usually so mild mannered, there was something different about Erika this morning. On this occasion she wasn't smiling. She was furious that the media attention we were attracting would backfire and she would have a problem with the authorities who were already 'gunning' for her.

When she spoke, the room went completely silent. Simon turned white with shock. Erika noticed.

"Oh Simon don't worry, you will have your death," she said softly "I'm just so cross."

We had to explain that the story of Simon attending the clinic had, we think, been leaked. We knew where the leak had come from. A campaigner had asked to make a film of Simon and I explaining our situation and Simon expressing his wish to die. I had called to tell him confidentially that Simon had decided to end his life early. He had asked to share the story. I clearly said no. He called later to say that a "work experience person" had accidentally leaked the story. I've no idea if that's true but I don't care either. Leaking our story was not the right or a kind thing to do. And it adds to my sense that assisted dying has become such a binary campaign message that the nuances and humanity of people's lives get lost along the way. My view was that some of the campaigners I met seemed to think that the end justified any means even if that meant trampling over people's lives.

To be fair Simon had also posted his intentions with a 'Goodbye world' message on LinkedIn. Although would the media really have found this alone? I doubt it.

None of this really mattered. And the one thing I have learnt through all my challenges is to choose one's fights. And this one was definitely in the not important enough category. Most importantly, Simon seemed to lap up the attention. He was one of the most open, gregarious people I've ever met. He relished the odd, the bizarre and the completely crazy. He genuinely could not give a stuff about what anybody else thought of him. He was a brilliant, loyal friend and a terrible enemy. He was tough and resilient so none of this behaviour really touched him.

He was also surrounded by people who loved him and would have fought tooth and nail to protect him. He knew that he was extraordinarily lucky in so many ways and he worried, as do I, how somebody in less advantageous situations may have coped.

***

Simon lay on the bed. I think it was a hospital bed. It was fine. Plain sheets, quite clinical but ok. My gaze was instantly drawn to the stand by the side of the bed. Above that dangled the thing we'd come for - the innocuous looking liquid that would kill my husband. Suddenly Simon started fumbling around looking for something. We all jumped up, desperate to help. Had he suddenly changed his mind? Did he want something? How could we help? "Mmmmmm," his voice was more of a constant mumble now. I got the word "phone" out of it. What in the world would he need his 'phone for? A moment of marital irritation flashed through my mind and a little reminder of how he'd driven me mad by always being on his mobile. How I would miss those every day irritations. Whatever did he want with it now?

But who were we to judge. It suddenly appeared. Was it in a coat pocket? Just cannot remember. But there it was and he was insistent. He fumbled about for what was probably minutes, but felt like hours. Suddenly my daughters' voices broke through the deafening silence. He'd written me a final message and got the girls to record it. I knew that my tears had distressed him, so I'd been bottling them up so tightly. But now they just fell fast and furious. He explained again how he felt he'd had no choice. That life had been great, but it was over for him. That he felt we had said everything that needed saying and that this death was better than a sudden death like a car accident. I so appreciated him doing this.

He was pleased with himself that his final little act had gone well and had the desired effect - all of us trembling and torn apart by the thought of losing this very special man. He'd moved us one final time with a huge Binner gesture out of left field. Always out of left field. And he told me, what I already knew, we'd had a hell of a life together. And not everybody gets that kind of love story.

The girls had spoken the words in their little heartbroken voices. Their maturity and lack of their own self-pity and rage touched me. They were losing him too, but we seemed to join together instead of breaking apart. How had we helped to bring up two such wonderful young women? Never once did either of them flinch from anything that was asked of them. Their grace and stoicism seemed to belong to people much older. Neither of them ever asked "What about me?" - they just wanted to help him. I think we did a good enough job with those girls.

***

The message ended and Erika set up a camera. She explained that Simon needed to be filmed for legal reasons. To prove that it was he who released the syringe pump so that the poison could be poured into his veins before moving to his great big heart and causing its final ever beat. Boom, boom, boom.

I glanced around and saw cameras everywhere. Simon was unfazed and looked directly into the lens and smiled for his last shot. That image is freeze-framed in my mind. He looked so dignified, so ready to leave. Erika then gently explained that when he let go of the syringe, Simon would die. He nodded and smiled. Again seemingly so at peace, in charge until the very end. I knew my husband so well; the little tells that would break through when he was frightened, upset, anything. I remembered his face twitching in disbelief as the doctor had given him his diagnosis just earlier that same year. If I could have wrapped up all the pain and taken it for him I would have. He was stripped bare as the dreadful truth of what was ahead seemed to devour his whole body. It was the second saddest thing I had ever seen in my life. The first was Chloë.

He nodded and pushed the syringe into its final place. He grasped my hand and I felt every last bit of strength leave my body and my legs buckled. Mike held onto me like the brave friend he had come to be. Erika gently stroked Simon's forehead, just as I had stroked Chloë's. She murmured softy "It's ok Simon. It will all be ok."

It took a couple of minutes. It took a lifetime. I have no idea what was true. Even the Swiss clocks had stopped and time stayed suspended for a long while. What I do remember is the room suddenly losing oxygen, like a plane falling from the sky. I wanted to grab an oxygen mask, a prop of some sort, but nothing was there. Something huge left the room leaving an airless space around us. I gasped to catch my breath. Was that the soul leaving? I wondered. And Simon had had such a huge soul. If it was, it would have been right. The strength of that energy leaving an enormous void in the room. An enormous void in life.

***

What happened next was surreal. The police entered the room. Normal procedure of course. The Swiss do everything very, very well and we had been warned that they would appear to ensure all processes had been followed and nothing was amiss. They did their investigations and we sat silently. There was no energy left. We stayed whilst my dear husband's empty body was lifted into a box and then disappeared into the cold, crisp Basel morning. It was still early I think.

We were all completely exhausted. I had, sadly, known that exhaustion before. When my daughter died. Holding all of the tears, anger, rage, hurt, yearning – all of it - tightly within so as not to upset that precious person… and then it could all come out as they left. But instead, with Simon, as with Chloë, it wasn't there anymore. I just felt a big empty vacuum.

We followed Erika to a cafe. How normal! A cafe. We even drank coffee together. And now the dream takes over. Somehow we got from the cafe to a boat. I even took a photo. There we all are taking a boat trip. Whatever were we thinking? We went to a restaurant. Wine and beer numbed us for a while. We'd deliberately planned not to stay too long in Basel and had an afternoon flight so next stop, the airport.

Simon's wheelchair! There it was. Huge, daunting, immoveable and empty. So very empty. It was NHS property, it had to go back. I clung tightly onto the chair feeling the last bits of my husband/my life falling away from me. On the plane. Don't remember a thing. A blur until the airport. Defeated, exhausted, not thinking straight we wandered out through the arrivals at Gatwick, wheelchair in tow. It was only later I realised what this would have looked like to the friends and family that came to greet us and cover us again with the warmth and love of people who cared very much about each other. Sian later told me of the shock that she felt as the Binner wheelchair, in all its glory, emerged through the gates. Its owner no longer in our world.

*****

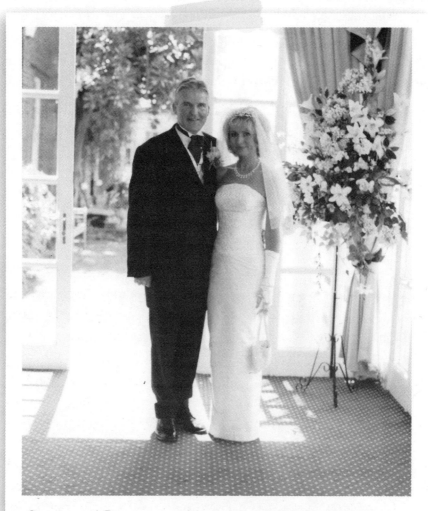

Simon and I on our wedding day, one of the happiest days of my life. I was so certain we'd grow old together...

TWO

'And when great souls die, after a period peace blooms, slowly and always irregularly. Spaces fill with a kind of soothing electric vibration. Our senses, restored, never to be the same, whisper to us. They existed. They existed. We can be. Be and be better. For they existed.' — Maya Angelou

THE DARK DAYS OF LIFE AFTER DEATH

THERE were many very dark days after Simon died. The film crew went away and I went back to the house we'd shared for 14 years. Thank goodness for Ralph the dog. The best golden retriever in the world who was, as always, delighted to have me back. But most importantly, thank God for Hannah and my two little grandchildren. The most perfect little beings who would grow up without really knowing how fabulous Simon and Chloë really were. And how much they would have loved them.

I can hardly bear to remember Simon sitting so proudly with Roman teaching him maths equations. "Simon, he's not even a year old," I'd protest. "Never too early to learn. He doesn't want to fall behind." Even though he was really a step-grandad, he insisted that the children drop the 'step' bit. "I've earned my place," he'd say proudly. Simon loved children. "I'm good with children and old people," he'd announce cherrily. "It's the ones in between that I have trouble with."

Children. Those special little beings. So innocent. Those huge eyes looking at you. Willing you to be ok. Telling you that life goes on. They need you.

In all my trials I've found that having a loving family and close friendship bonds around you is as good as it will ever get. I don't think they have to be blood related. Just the people you know are in your tribe. The ones you sit around doing nothing with. The ones that make your heart sing. The ones that walk beside you. The ones who have your back whatever, wherever.

The mind is such a wonderful thing it seems to block out the days of greatest pain. But there were some. My daughter Hannah had moved in with me. It was a lifeline for both of us, I think. I had to be ok. My daughter deserved the best mother she could have. She'd been through so much and she was still only 22. In those early days she was my very reason for living. My only reason. I really didn't see any point in anything. Why had life been so cruel? I'm not one to wallow in self-pity. It's an emotion I've always disliked in others as well as in myself. But I felt sore, raw and deflated and couldn't help the occasional, well maybe more than occasional, wail of "WHY ME!"

I'm sure that a psychotherapist could have had a field day with my family. Over ambitious mother. Blended family. Youngest girl gets ill and dies. Oldest girl feels she needs to build the little broken family again. Drops out of education – time for that later – and brings firstly Roman into our lives while Chloë was still ill. Ah Roman he has the smell of Chloë on him. She touched him. She loved him. He knew her as present. And then some nine months after Chloë died little Nahla popped out. A girl. What a gift. If anybody had said she was there to replace Chloë I would have punched them. I really would. Nothing could, ever. But it was really nice that she was a girl. Half Turkish, a quarter Irish, she looked like a little coffee bean with those huge saucer eyes. Hannah and I had inherited the milk-white skin and freckles of our Celtic ancestry. We were both so enchanted by the olive skin and chestnut brown eyes of our two little additions.

At the time it could have all looked like a huge disaster. My super bright Hannah ditches the chance of university and the life I'd been planning for her since she first came blinking into my world. Instead she has two children and becomes a single mum in her early 20s. Not exactly what was in the life plan of an uber ambitious Mother.

But life has the strangest way of playing with us don't you think. What could have been a disaster became exactly the opposite – for all of us really. New life; a whole new reason to get up, get going and make things happen. If anybody knew how precious a minute with a child was, it was us. We had to buck up and try again to build that perfect existence that we had once enjoyed. How sad that we didn't realise just how blessed we were back then. We were all somehow being given a second chance now. Two new beings here. Get up, there's work to do.

But my wise husband had understood this early. A dear friend reminded me just the other day how Simon had sent one of his daft quizzes out to friends and family. This was just the kind of thing he was always doing. Playing tricks on us all, obscure puzzles, always getting us guessing about something or other. The quiz had been about Hannah, can't remember the detail, but the answer was that Hannah was pregnant. He was so proud that she was pregnant. He'd told that same friend that I couldn't bring myself to tell anybody, as I was just coming to terms with it myself. But he was delighted. He verbalised what I could never do. He told her he didn't know how much longer that Chloë would be with us and he knew the devastation that this would cause to all of us. A new baby in the family wouldn't replace anything, but would be essential in enabling us to go on. How prophetic he was.

Roman was and is a very special child to us for many reasons. His birth seemed almost biblical in its power. A dying child. A newborn baby. It was as if God was saying well you can't give up now can you. Look at this perfection. You have to dust yourselves off and open those weary hearts again. This child needs you all and he needs you in good shape.

I so hope that boy grows up to have the most glorious life. If

Hannah and I have anything to do with it he will. And little Nahla Chloë too. Hannah was right not naming her Chloë, although I would have loved it so much at the time. She wasn't Chloë, Chloë was dead and gone by the time that Nahla was born… She was – is – Nahla, her own unique little being who will grow to be the woman she wants to be. Secretly I love the fact that she has something of Chloë about her, not just her middle name. A sunny confidence that allows her to glide above ordinary life, a real delight in the world and, of course, she's a beautiful little thing too.

Looking back I was terrified that Hannah's chosen path would destroy any chance she had of having a good, happy future. Through my own troubles my education and my career provided the platform

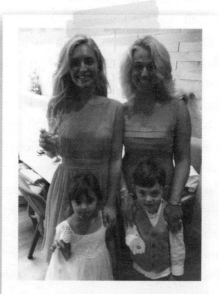

Me, Hannah and my beautiful grandchildren, Roman and Nahla Chloë

for hope. When life got hard I just worked harder. And that paid off. Work was safe for me; I saw a clear equation between the effort that was put in and the subsequent success, promotion and finances. It was so wonderfully structured. I wanted Hannah to have the same thing. But she isn't me. She has her own unique qualities of which I need to constantly remind myself when interfering Mum mode takes over. She has her own path to follow. I see that now and it has allowed me to kick back and enjoy our little family in a whole new and different way.

The lens we choose to see life through is all, I believe. The thing I'd labelled a disaster and a demonstration to the world of what a rubbish mother I'd been to her, turned out to be the best thing that could have happened. To us all.

Hannah, who was far too bright and accomplished for her own good, was also wild and at times self-destructive. Feisty, determined and so very brave, she was hard to handle as a teenager and I fear my own inability to cope with her had squashed her in some ways.

What a waste of energy all that worry was! Her 'wildness' and inability to conform are the qualities that enabled her to not only survive losing a sister, a beloved stepfather and single parenthood but catapulted her into a separate universe. Simon, in his wisdom, had spotted her talent and resilience very early. He handpicked her to take over his healthcare company, overlooking me for the job. Which was a very good decision in hindsight!

He gave her the reins and boy did she fly. A young woman of 23, with no real commercial experience – oh and two small children – she took on the company. It was really, really tough on her, but it also made her. In the years since Simon died she has turned the company around and carved out a fantastic reputation as an ethical, dynamic local businesswoman. Recognition has come thick and fast and she's scooping up national business awards. One after the other.

She is also the most fantastic mother and daughter. It reminds me of something Simon's father had said. A working class man who'd defied all the odds and got not one, but two, first class degrees at Cambridge he always feared that Simon would be 'deprived of being deprived.' He was tough on Simon, refusing to give him any funding after his own engineering degree, also at Cambridge. It had been hard for Simon at the time but he'd grown to respect his father for what he saw as a 'gift.' It enabled him to carve his own path, to be his own man.

Hannah's life had been scarred, or so I thought, by my separation from her father and so much loss. Would she always have made a success of life just on her own terms, or did these difficulties help her to dig deep, to show a bit more courage, more resilience because there really was no safety net? Nobody can answer this. What I do know is that she has soared, where she could have crashed. And for this I am so full of admiration and gratitude.

Believe me I wouldn't wish what happened to us on anybody. But I

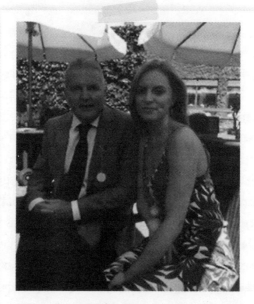

Simon and Hannah enjoying a day out at Wimbledon

do believe, begrudgingly, that the only good thing to come out of our turmoil is an iron will not to let it drown us. I notice in my daughter something that's also in me. It's a fire in the belly to keep on fighting. To recognise that life can be incredibly tough, but the trick is to keep on getting up again and again. And if necessary again after that. I cannot believe that anything can hurt me again as much as watching my baby girl, as that is what she was to me, fight cancer and succumb to it. The only positive is that I now have a strange fearless freedom. I don't fear the same things that I used to. I seem to have accepted at the deepest level that we have so little control over anything at all in reality. We may as well kick back and enjoy the ride. I came to the point where I knew there was a clear decision: a lovely joyful loving life or a bitter, long painful life. I chose the first and I know this is what Chloë and Simon would have wanted.

***

But back to widowhood. It's a unique loss. Not like losing a child. Nothing is. It sounds brutal but the truth is however much you loved your spouse or your partner, you can get another one if you want. I dispute strongly that this makes your love any less or the pain any easier. It is just a fact. I loved Simon dearly and because of that I know I can love somebody else again. I loved being married and because of that, I know that I could marry again. I've never stopped loving Simon and never will. I have no wish to become some kind of Miss Havisham character. When somebody dies the relationship keeps evolving if you let it. You can't love them in the same way, but they remain deep in your heart if you keep it open enough. I even still get cross with Simon sometimes and would you believe even now, I run over some of the arguments we had in my head and try and prove that I was right. That makes me smile. He would have loved that and said something like, "For Christ's sake can't you drop this now I'm dead!" He had the most wonderful sense of humour, a little too black at times as nothing was off limits, but he was so very, very funny. Gosh I do miss that. We had this magic together.

Like me with Chloë, Simon's mother quite rightly said she can never replace her son. However old that child is the pain is inordinate and so out of the natural order of what we expect the world to deliver to us. A child can never replace the parent that is lost. And for that reason, for me at least, it is a unique loss and so very sad but in the hierarchy of loss, if there is such a thing, it isn't the worst.

But being widowed does have very unique difficulties. And it's

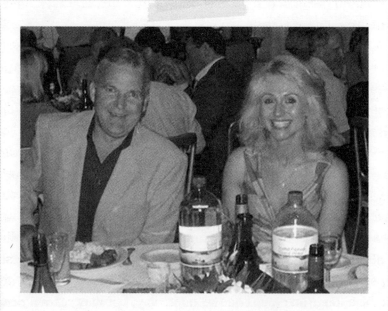

At a dinner – Simon and I shared a
love of socialising

because I had such a brilliant – not perfect – but pretty good marriage that I have subsequently wanted to form another relationship. Simon and I discussed this and he gave me his blessing. In hindsight this is such a generous, kind thing to have done. My life afterwards would have been more challenging if he hadn't. I would have felt far more guilt. As it was I knew, as I started to heal, I had so much life force left, so much love to give, I wanted to share my life with somebody again. I'm so glad that we discussed this.

I recall at this moment how my husband, who as you probably get by now, was rather gloriously bonkers, decided one morning that I would not be able to cope on my own. It wasn't true. I'd coped with the loss of Chloë; nothing could ever be more difficult than that. But I played along. I believe that he wanted to remind me how very important he was and that I would fall apart without him. What did he do? A northerner, Simon was very pragmatic. Describing himself as a 'worn out old car,' he said, "It's time for a new one." So he wrote a glowing testimonial of his 'wonderful wife' and tried to put me on the dating site Match.com.

'One wife available. Well tested and highly recommended. Not a very good driver, but skilled in the kitchen…' In typical nutty Simon style he imagined himself as the sole occupant of the 'husband interview panel.' He thought it was a brilliant idea. He could leave me with a handpicked husband to take over his role.

Needless to say I was horrified. But, like everything Simon did, it was also extremely funny. And if I was honest I had flirted with the idea, so very briefly, of a life after Simon. At 50 I knew that there could be a long time left. I had wondered if I could ever love another person one day but never in a million years would I have shared that thought. Simon, practical as ever, put the plan in action.

Very wisely Match.com wrote a lovely letter back saying that they were terribly sorry for the situation we found ourselves in but posting such an advertisement was a breach of their code of conduct – namely that husbands who still existed could not advertise their wife to other single men! Priceless.

I have to say I soon found this whole escapade hilarious. Black humour had become very much part of our life. It had to; we needed to laugh sometimes. It was one of the reasons that Simon and I worked so well together. We shared this rather off-centre sense of humour. We also liked to push at boundaries together. Do weird and wonderful things whenever possible – llama walks, treasure hunts that led to friends being apprehended by the police as the clues would lead to people's gardens, life coaching holidays…we shared a belief that we needed to jump into life and bounce around in everything it had to offer. I think it's fair to say we lived a very full life and that's a very good thing to look back on.

***

I remember tender moments, such as after a particularly distressing emotional breakdown. Unsurprisingly Simon would sometimes plunge into the most catastrophic despair. Unable to speak, the pain seemed to be stuck inside him pushing at every pore to come out. I remember the first time this had happened. I'd been out at a yoga class. We had the most delightful Scottish children's nanny staying with us. Her name was Jennie and she had formerly been an air stewardess. She was great in a crisis and implanted herself as a key member of Simon's support team; as well as looking after the children. I came back in the door one evening. Simon had been his usual jovial self when I left, but I walked into a black mood hanging heavy in the house. And then I saw the most pitiful sight ever: my husband sobbing his heart out. Jennie's face was drained of colour as she looked desperately at me from the sitting room doorway. She'd been trying so hard to calm him for what I later found out had been hours. I joined her and we held him tight. It was terrible. He had no voice, so he couldn't tell us what he was thinking, feeling. It seemed that all the pain and anguish were trapped inside of him and he couldn't get them out. It was a horrible, horrible evening. We were all traumatised. It seemed to go on for hours more. We stroked his head, held him and tried to speak gently, promising him everything would be ok. But it was so far from being ok.

***

I had always thought that physical pain was the most frightening thing. But now I don't. But that is absolutely no consolation. That feeling of being locked in, unable to communicate, to control any aspect of your body or your life. Of things getting worse and worse, but your mind and brain stay as alert as ever. No pain killing drugs to dull the emotional as well as the physical agony. You are just left in a body that is falling apart. That is surely the worst it gets.

We were all coming to the end of our resources. We were all so tired. Later a 20mg daily dose of the antidepressant citalopram dulled these episodes. This made it easier for the people around him. But I'm not entirely convinced that it made things better for Simon. Jennie and I were deeply shaken by the incident, but the next day he was up and dressed again making his usual silly jokes – on paper of course as that was the only way left for him to communicate. Did these breakdowns act as some kind of release for him? God knows that he needed some kind of vent for all the emotion that was building within him; something had to give. It's impossible to convey how utterly heart breaking it is to watch a big proud man reduced to a sobbing wreck. It is, after cancer in a child, the most horrifying thing I have witnessed in my entire life.

***

Simon and I discussed his death. He was clear he felt it was his life and whilst he cared about my view, at the end of the day it was he who would decide. He was clear he knew he'd had a really good life. He'd started in a loving family, was super bright and had all of the best opportunities. He loved his family and had loads of friends. He admitted sometimes to being so furious that he'd finally found something he really liked doing – running his own business and doing something purposeful – and wished he'd done it earlier. He was so cross that he'd wasted time "being a bit depressed" or not appreciating how "bloody lucky" he was. But I really think he was generally ok about how he'd lived his life. He had a very clear code of conduct, strong values and, as a friend had said, "His moral compass was always pointed in the right direction." He never swerved away from what he thought was right and I think that gave him some kind of peace.

Simon knew very well what I thought of him. After Chloë I have never wasted opportunities to tell people what they mean to me. He knew I'd had a tough life and I think he enjoyed his role in what he described as my "knight in shining armour." And that's what he was to me.

I was, I am, a strong person. I have survived so much. But part of being strong is admitting when you are terrified. I was utterly terrified of losing my husband. I tried not to think about this at the time as I didn't want to transfer this fear to him and add any more to his burden. I wanted him to feel loved so much, but not to worry that I would fall apart.

He spoke sadly, wistfully about Chloë and said how much he'd loved her and the other girls. He recalled a very special moment when Chloë had called him over. She was dying. She had a bumpy relationship with Simon, but she knew he loved her. He loved her like a daughter. And that is the best gift you can give to a stepchild. She took his hand and looked into his eyes and simply said, "Thank you Simon." He was distraught that he hadn't managed to say anything back. He was so surprised by the gesture and hadn't wanted to let on that he knew that she was dying. It played on his mind and there was nothing he could do now.

***

Simon did not believe that he would see any of us again, and he said he was so sad he hadn't seized the moment with Chloë and told her that one of his main regrets in life was that Hannah and Chloë hadn't had been his own children. I really don't think he needed to worry. I believe that they both knew that. His actions spoke way louder than any words he could have uttered. He had no religion and to him there was no God, no afterlife. "This is it. The end." I admired his pragmatism and the fact he held true to his beliefs; but it felt harsh and blunt to me. I wanted to believe something. I wanted to believe that we might meet again somewhere, but he would have seen that as weak, fanciful thinking.

I'm glad that he knew that we all would have cared for him. And with so much love around him he would have got the best care ever. I think he appreciated that and was slightly surprised. "I thought the last thing you'd want is to care for someone else," he wrote one morning. And then with love: "I want you to have a life. You've had enough care and pain. I don't want you to have to do that for me. I don't want you to see me like this."

As time moves on I understand this better. At the time I wanted him to live in whatever condition. I would have sorted it. I always did. But I cannot deny that it would have been incredibly difficult for all of us. I cannot lie about this. Care up close is really hard. I think in his actions he saved us all from this. From the burden. I would have taken on that burden though and with a glad heart, but the decision wasn't mine, it was all Simon's. I think we both really meant it when we said "In sickness and in health." But I was not deluded. People who care for others have a hugely difficult time. You don't realise until you get

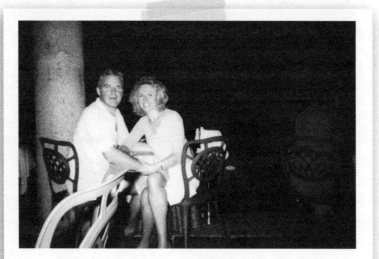

At the start of our wonderful married life.
Honeymooning in Italy

there that actually there isn't nearly enough help to go around. So often it is the relatives and friends who shoulder a very hefty workload. I'm really glad that we had the time to have these difficult conversations. We came from opposing sides, but we stated our case, we listened respectfully, disagreed but, and this is so important for the life after death, we carried on loving each other.

And I do carry on loving him. More faintly now, but more deeply. I often wonder what his view would be on all the crazy politics of today. He would have loved the Trump story and been hugely amusing in his reflections. I keep Chloë and Simon's ashes in my wardrobe. They seem to belong there. I don't know why I don't scatter them or make some memorial for them. But I don't. I feel they would be too far away from me and too cold in the earth. I feel I've done a decent job of trying to move on, but I can't let this one go. Am I being selfish? I'm sure that others may want a grave stone to visit. But it seems too difficult a choice for me. For now I keep them close, right in the midst of all my things. Right with me. They were my little family. It was so lovely for a while. When I remember something annoying that Simon had done I give the ashes a good shake. How he would laugh if he could see me. "Never speak in hushed tones about me," he ordered. "I was a difficult, annoying bugger and you need to remember me how I was. It's disrespectful to paint me as some kind of saint." And he'd always add: "And don't you dare have some park bench named in my honour. I'll come and haunt you if you do."

***

THE WHITE FURY OF GRIEF

CS Lewis says grief feels like fear. I get that, but it doesn't nearly cover it all. For me the anger has been one of the most difficult things to bear. Fear is socially acceptable, anger isn't so much. Elisabeth Kübler-Ross, the Swiss American psychiatrist and author of the groundbreaking book *On Death and Dying* (1969) introduced us to the model of the five stages of grief: denial, anger, bargaining, depression and acceptance. Later in her life she added that the stages did not follow a chronological order and that a person could get stuck in one stage or move backwards and forwards between many.

I have been shocked at how much anger has figured in my journey. And not an anger I felt before. This is cold white fury that could destroy anything in its wake.

There are, I have found, many dangers here. Bury it and its ferocity could cause the most severe depression – after all the experts warn us that anger turned inwards leads to depression. Focus it outwards and God knows what could happen – untethered it could destroy anything, everything in its path.

To God, if one believes in such a thing. To doctors who can't cure your loved one. To the friend who unwittingly says the wrong thing (be kind and patient with friends; we have no idea what they are going through too). I have found two ways of dealing with this. The first is writing, writing and writing. Trying to hold on to the emotion and placing it for scrutiny on the paper before taking any action. Setting all those horrid, nasty, ugly thoughts down. We all have them. How could we not in this hurly burly difficult world.

Secondly, imagery is great for defusing the strength of the emotion. Take the anger out an innate object well away from you and far from other people. Fire off all those thoughts towards this place and build your own bonfire. You can then literally set fire to it in your mind. The thoughts no longer festering in your body but not hurting anybody else either.

It works. Sometimes.

I promised you I'd tell the truth so here is my abridged version of some of my angry thoughts:

I am absolutely fuming that my husband left me to fend in this world alone. That was not the deal. I counted his calories, made him walk, run, dealt with his medical appointments, cooked him fine organic meals, reduced his stress levels, cared about him, loved him, cherished him. BUT it wasn't enough. I wasn't enough. All my love, with all my heart was pointless and useless in the face of MND.

Was it arrogant of me to think that everything that I had to offer would stop Simon wanting to die?

The moments we lay together were quite beautiful in their darkness. We'd started together with such promise. Already in mid-life – me 36 him 42 – we'd had a chance to start again. But at this point we were recognising that our life and love were running out and we all die alone.

I was heartbroken and furious that this wasn't enough for him. I know that sounds crass, arrogant, selfish…but we human beings are flawed. I think about this issue often. In the heat of battle I was a brilliant warrior – I was great in a fight; it's the quiet and silence I struggle with. I was not thinking so much about Simon and what he really wanted. And could it be this reason, more than any other, that I have avoided the assisted dying debate? I am an unreliable witness as I had such a vested interest in my husband being alive for my own well-being.

On the other side of things Simon was, quite possibly, acting selfishly too. He was so traumatised by this dreadful illness he could only think of what he needed. Don't we all revert to the worst versions of ourselves under pressure? He wanted out and my and our family's love for him became a barrier to what he wanted. Sure he would have hated it any other way and he knew how blessed he was to be so adored. But it was definitely a dilemma for him. He wanted to die and this pesky wife of his was pleading with him to live.

How very different from the slippery slope argument that people who don't agree with assisted dying often cite: that relatives will be relieved that their own lives aren't curtailed too much by having to look after a disabled relative. Or that precious resources are flying out the door to pay the ever increasing cost of care.

Like most situations ours was unique. It didn't fit the usual stereotypes. To me it goes to show how difficult it is to make a binary argument for or against assisted dying. There are so many different shades of grey. It's a massively complicated issue.

***

Straight after Simon's death I squirmed when people, sometimes quite forcefully, pushed their view of my husband's death onto me. Some said that they were pleased that Simon had got his wish and what a wonderful thing it was that he'd done. We'd opened our lives up to national and international scrutiny – the film was apparently very popular in China – why ever was I surprised that people had a view?

But I really hated hearing this. I wasn't ready to hear this. I was especially furious with the people who seemed to want to continually convince me that he'd done the right thing. This was entirely different from the friends who have thought carefully about the issue and believe that we should allow assisted dying in our country to avoid unnecessary suffering. This includes some of the friends that went to Switzerland with us. They too have seen this thing up close. I totally respect that view. But the people who thought it was their duty to convince me; how did they know!! I found this attitude insensitive at best and offensive at worst. I hope not to treat others like this. We are all so different and come to issues from different places. Heavens, I don't really, truly understand my own feelings and know that they sometimes seem so conflicted. I'm suspicious of people who think they have all the answers, know all the truths. We all have our own truth and this, to me, is the most important thing to hold onto. I love debate, thoughtful, considered debate but please, please keep me away from the know it all zealots. I want nothing to do with them.

More recently I was touched by a message that Rowan Deacon the director of the BBC film sent me. She'd been at an academic conference in Switzerland where they'd been debating assisted dying. She relayed a discussion between a psychiatrist and a theologian. The psychiatrist had been most interested in Simon's character. No surprises there! He felt his unique character and his way of looking at the world led and shaped his end. The theologian said gently, "The wife! Nobody is listening to the wife."

I loved hearing that. It endorsed me. I had always felt like a lone voice. I didn't have a religious argument to hide behind or bolster me. I wasn't arguing against assisted dying for any religious reason at all. I was arguing from deep in my soul. Something didn't sit right. Hearing of this man's voice helped me to feel that I had a right. I wasn't sure of that before. I had a right to feel differently. Differently from my husband, from most, if not all, of our friends but definitely from my husband. I wasn't just being selfish. I was, I hope, speaking my truth. As Simon hoped that his story would help others in his situation, I hope mine may help others in mine. The wives, the partners, the family members who just aren't sure. Who are left wondering did we really all do enough for him, to make his life matter whatever the circumstances. I am left feeling that an assisted death leaves its very own unpredictable marks. I cannot help but think that the chances of complicated grief, after such an event, are that much more likely. I think it's difficult to come to terms with.

I would have found it much harder to live afterwards if I had readily followed the consensus and supported Simon wholeheartedly. At times I felt extremely pressurised to go with the flow. But I've learnt over the years that I have a steely will that just won't be hushed. I spoke my truth. It didn't matter that people couldn't hear it. It mattered very much to me. And it did matter that Simon knew that I would love him come what may. I wasn't going anywhere and I certainly was not looking at an alternative future with rose tinted spectacles. I knew that whatever path we chose it would be difficult.

In truth pre-Simon I would have joined the assisted dying debate with my usual campaigning spirit. Pontificating about how I would feel in any given situation. But this was different. This was not some theoretical discussion. This was my man. My life. My loss.

***

THE LONELY WOOD OF WIDOWHOOD

A dear friend Heather gave me the best advice She'd lost a child too. She knew pain. How do I go on? I begged her to give me an answer. "You get up, you put one foot in front of the other. And then when you make it to the end of the day you give yourself a huge hug for making it through."

Friends were wonderful. At first I didn't feel any of the isolation of being left out by other couples that is apparently so common in widowhood. They invited me everywhere and I tried really hard to go. But it was difficult.

I'd been so independent as a young woman. From early on I'd never flinched at the idea of going anywhere alone. I'd never felt uncomfortable alone at social gatherings. I always just saw it as an opportunity to meet new and interesting people. I was therefore really surprised to be hit by a crippling social anxiety when Simon died. He and I had been part of a strong friendship group. We holidayed together, ate together, partied together. Later we buried first my child and then my husband together. They'd been part of my life for so long, but I felt myself wanting to hide away. Every time I went anywhere I could see my hands trembling and felt that I'd had a layer of skin ripped away. I'd always try and turn up, but the tears would be so near the surface I would often leave early. I would go home alone, gazing in the mirror; a haunted, gaunt face which said, "Please no more," stared back at me...

In hindsight I wish I hadn't tried so hard. People would have understood. What I really needed to do was to hide away for a while and nurse my wounds. I had a dream once that I retreated to a deep dark wood and just sat and contemplated what had happened. Far from being a frightening place it became the place I sought solace. It was in my mind, of course, but I still retreat there. I call it my lonely wood of widowhood. I just couldn't cope with any human interaction. I needed time alone to meditate on the memories, the great times we'd had together, the fact that I was now different, not like them anymore. I was a widow and this would take a huge adjustment. It was far bigger than I ever imagined it would be and way more painful. I wasn't myself any longer and that was going to take some getting used to.

A few months after Simon's death I wrote my widow's five tips for survival:

1. Stay connected with people you love. If you can't make it to a party, send a text. You will be left out of things; it's just the way life is. Things have changed. Try not to take this personally and just keep connecting - eventually you will want to return to a social life and good friends take years to make so don't let them slip away. When somebody dies we are all extremely raw and vulnerable. It's so easy to hurt each other as we have a thinner skin. Stay kind, stay gentle, stay connected.

2. Take the lead. I was 50 when I was widowed. I knew only one other woman who'd been widowed. Friends don't know what to do or say. They haven't been there and until you have you really can't know. I will share my story, but my whole narrative is different and makes me who I am. Advice is rarely useful. A listening ear, a touch of a hand, a hug, these all really matter. I know you may be flat out on the floor but keep up the conversations and tell people what you need and what you want. Some may run for the hills; most won't. Others will really surprise you with their kindness. And in the midst of all this there is the opportunity to make new deeper bonds too. You are different; a new you. This can be strangely exciting and lead to new opportunities. Grab them, life is way too short not to.

3. Look for another partner when/if YOU are ready. Only you will know this. Be kind, but firm, with others. Other people will be grieving too, and they may not be ready to let you move on. This is your life and you only get one chance. There is no right time; only the right time for you.

4. Cry, cry, cry. Scream, scream, scream. Write, write, write. Embrace the emotion and get it out there. You may well, like me, have lost the love of your life. It's so unfair so shout about it. Trapped emotion leads to depression.

5. Get a dog if this is possible for your domestic set up. Nothing

beats that wagging tail and the fact that they know exactly when to snuggle up next to you when the tears start. No words are necessary and sometimes that is the most helpful thing of all.

And be kind to yourself. You are so fragile; you need care and lots of it. Don't expect others to be the sole providers of this. They will for a while, but they have their own stuff, their own lives going on. Take on the role as your own primary care giver. Do whatever you need to feel better - finances allowing - take up that new hobby, something you've never dared to do before. Embrace that freedom and start a whole new life story. Celebrate your love but build on from it.

*****

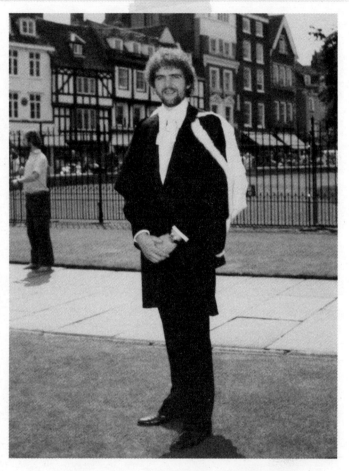

Simon as a Cambridge undergrad

THREE

"It is not death that a man should fear, but he should fear never beginning to live."
- Marcus Aurelius

WHOSE LIFE IS IT ANYWAY?

I HAVE steered clear of campaigning for a change in the law on assisted dying, despite being asked many times. I feel I cop out of the argument but, unusually for me, I remain ambivalent about this situation. My biggest fear being the slippery slope of a lack of value on life and the fact that many people in my husband's position may feel more of a burden than they already do.

I have instead tried to show on as many occasions as possible - including talks to schools with the most wonderful curious young people - the up close and personal picture of what assisted dying actually looks like and the unique scars that it leaves behind. I think that this second point has not been considered well enough. There are scars for children here too. And these can linger for many years.

If pushed to decide one way or the other, I'm swayed mostly by the argument that we should not be outsourcing our compassion to another country. Nor should we be allowing it as an option only to pointy-elbowed, middle class people who can afford the fee.

I kick mostly against the binary argument which seems way too stark. On one side they scream, "Legalise assisted dying now" and on the other, "Tighten the law and ensure it stays illegal." In the infamous words of the author and scientist Ben Goldacre (he was referring to issues around medical research and the pharmaceutical industry), "I think you'll find it's a bit more complicated than that."

The firm that Simon founded, and Hannah now runs, is a healthcare company offering services to people with long-term health conditions or coming to the end of their lives. Care at this level is expensive. It is very labour intensive and is heavily dependent on providing the right people and the right training. Robust regulation is essential as is continuing monitoring. It all costs a lot of money.

We see for ourselves on a daily basis how people can suffer in the last stages of their lives. Yet still I think one of the greatest miseries as people get older is the loneliness. And would we ever allow a law that allowed people to kill themselves because no one wanted to visit them? That may sound simplistic but ask anybody who works with the elderly and infirm and they will tell you about the pernicious nature of people who have nobody to bother with them.

I witness firsthand how older people in particular can feel a burden. There's a sense that they don't deserve all the care and attention. They want younger people to have it. That said, I also see the wonder of families who would do anything possible to make their relative comfortable. Of staff who dedicate their lives to genuinely caring for these people as if they were members of their own families. I see the value and purpose that these people get. Far away from the news headlines that scream about elder abuse, I have been stunned by a far more usual attitude of deep love and compassion for people coming to the end of their lives. When a client dies, the whole company seems to mourn as if a much loved family member has left the room and I believe that we all feel a little more connected, a little closer because of what we have witnessed. It helps with that sense of community. Again, this is not a black and white argument.

There are some neurological diseases, like MND, that seem beyond human endurance. And yet we know that most people, even with these diseases, don't choose to kill themselves. The inequality of the current system rankles with me most. Whilst the law seems to turn a blind eye to it, it will act if somebody tries to fundraise to help somebody go. If you are poor and or don't have relatives or friends to help you, well tough luck, it's down to the NHS. And the NHS, while so wonderful in so many ways, is pretty useless when it comes to these rare untreatable illnesses.

I do not by any means believe that there is sanctity or honour in suffering and I'm eternally grateful for the wonderful hardcore drugs that largely alleviated the physical pain of Chloë's cancer. But there is a humility, dignity and value in staying, caring and watching as our loved ones die. Letting go of the absurd belief that we control anything at all and just being with the person we love as the process of death takes hold.

In her deeply moving book *With the End in Mind*, palliative medicine pioneer Dr Kathryn Mannix makes the case for 'the therapeutic power of approaching death not with trepidation, but with openness, clarity, and understanding.' Her agenda is quite obviously making the case for better end of life care. She urges us all to make friends with death as she sees it as the biggest taboo in our society and the only certainty we all share. Through 30-odd stories of normal humans, dying normal deaths, she shows how the dying embrace living not because they are unusual or brave, but because that is what we humans do.

She takes us on a journey of her patients and allows us to sit by their bedsides with her as they die. I was especially touched by the story of Ujjal, a Dutchman in his 30s who had been diagnosed with cancer of the rectum. The side effects make for horrendous reading and one could easily see how one would rather die than go through the horror and indignities of these. But when he came to it he didn't want to. He didn't want the certainty of death; he wanted the uncertainty of hope. He was terminally ill and assisted dying is legal in the Netherlands for all the right reasons. But this man eventually fled to the UK to die in a hospice here as he felt pressurised by the constant – and definitely kindly – offers of a way out of his pain.

As Dr Mannix points out: 'The possibility of unintended pressure is a dilemma currently confronting healthcare systems across the world. Once the euthanasia genie is out of the bottle, you must be careful what you wish for.'

(Just for clarity here there is a difference between assisted dying and euthanasia. Doctor-assisted dying refers to the physician providing the means for death, most often with a prescription. Euthanasia means that the physician would act directly, for instance by giving a lethal injection, to end the patient's life.)

Another story from Mannix's book also resonated with me: 'Eric was a Head Teacher. With Capital letters. He was an organiser, a man who got things done.' (He sounded a similar alpha male character to my Simon. He too sounded a good man with a huge heart.) 'At first Eric was determined to go to Switzerland for an assisted death. But as time went on he worked with the doctors to adapt to each stage of the development of his illness. The doctors addressed his fears - such as choking to death - and gave hard evidence to allay some of them. Such as a recent case study of several hundred MND patients who were followed up until they died and precisely none of them died choking.' Mannix says that dying is usually far gentler than that.

Eric adapted and took joy in the simple things of life. Such a cliché I know, but my experience has been throughout the death of my child and my husband that it is the little things that matter so much; and that are so missed.

Eric lived to enjoy a Christmas with his family and then he decided he would stop his own antibiotics as he was ready to die. It struck me that there are many UK-based exit paths along the way in the progress of MND. He said he was glad he hadn't died earlier. "I would have missed so much. I had no idea that I would be able to tolerate living such a changed life." He added, "People need to understand this... I wanted to die before something happened that I couldn't bear. But I didn't die, and the thing I dreaded happened. But I found that I could bear it. I wanted euthanasia, and no one could do it. But if they hadn't then when would I have asked for it? Chances are I would have asked for it too early and I would have missed Christmas."

Like many people with MND, Eric succumbed to pneumonia - in my parents' day this was dubbed 'the old person's friend.' He slipped into unconsciousness and died peacefully.

Just one example, hence not statistically significant, I know. My husband was one example too.

Mannix, in her beautiful compassionate manner which seeps through the book, writes: 'The strength of the human spirit is astonishing. People all think that they have a limit, beyond which they cannot endure. Their capacity to adapt and to reset their limits has been a constant wonder to me over my decades in working with people living with some of the most challenging illnesses imaginable.'

***

As a palliative carer, Dr Mannix obviously comes from one side of the argument and this is just one story. As we know there have been several high profile campaigners in the UK who have fought tirelessly to be allowed to end their own lives as they feel they are experiencing intolerable suffering. I've seen that suffering and I really do get that.

I accept that the current situation is unclear and I know that my 'argument' if you can call it that is somewhat unfashionable in the circles in which I move. If you have enough money, good enough reasons, and enough 'balls' to go abroad and die in Switzerland – one of the few countries to accept foreigners into its assisted dying scheme – then you can. Although importantly you can never assume that and you do need to be ready for possibility of arrest or at least police questioning when you re-enter the UK. It is not for the faint hearted.

If you don't have enough money and try and fund raise your final trip (a pretty fair and creative way to sort this particular issue) the authorities are likely to come down on you like a ton of bricks. Sisters Tara O'Reilly and Rose Baker discovered this in 2015 when they organised a fundraiser to take their MND-stricken mother Jackie Baker to Dignitas. Following a complaint from Care not Killing, the anti-suicide organisation, two police officers visited the sisters and explained they could be prosecuted for abetting suicide if they didn't stop their actions. They stopped.

It's certainly a strange law…

***

If we make assisted dying legal do we not risk devaluing the already dubious value that we, as a society, put on the frail and infirm? I have a lot of faith in the next generation. Looking around at the young people I know I do see a shift towards a search for a better, kinder, more purposeful future. It was different in my day. I was starting out in the narcissistic 'loads of money' '80s and '90s. We thought that the fun would go on forever. But even so the fact that we in the UK share the values of the majority of other countries and don't allow assisted suicide says a lot about us. It says we care or at least are trying to care about people at every stage of their life. Yet it is interesting that surveys seem to show that the vast majority of people say they want assisted dying legalised in the UK, but it always seems to be voted down by Parliament…

The other day I read about a new invention launched at an international exhibition – a death capsule. People could just pop in and it would all be over. Sounds nuts now, but who knows in the future. Be careful what we wish for, I guess.

***

I went to the funeral recently of my friend's father. He was a Hindu and, by all accounts, quite a character. I loved the stories of his life, how he'd come from India as a young man and become a barrister in the UK. I watched this sad, but very uplifting ceremony of a man in his 80s who'd lived an amazing life. His two daughters and his seven grandchildren sobbing with love, tenderness and loss. They didn't care that he was old; they were distraught that he was gone. They just wanted a bit more time. It was beautiful to watch. Enriching and I felt everybody there felt a little bit better after being part of such an event full of the love of a family.

I have another friend who dedicated years of her life helping to care for her elderly mother who'd had a stroke. She was a busy business woman and worked full time, but she visited her mother almost every day. She bought her the finest Chanel perfumes, painted her nails bright pink and would more often than not bring her a fresh coffee in the morning and a sherry before bedtime. She often brought her out to dinner with us. I remember so well seeing her tenderly brushing her mother's hair, putting her lipstick on and then gently feeding her at our table as we all laughed and told cheeky jokes. Just girls together, young, old and middle-aged.

Enough already! I hear you shout. Life just isn't like that. Getting old is tough and people often just don't have enough time. And I think I do drive people crazy with my glass half full attitude to life. But my experiences have changed me at such a fundamental level. I have such a different view of what makes me happy. I take time now to care about the little things. I truly know how precious life is. I still crave those stylish new Russell and Bromley courts that will definitely change my life… And I adore clothes, obscenely expensive jewellery, fine wine, all of it and more. But I now realise that these are just the cherries on the top and wonderful if you have them but not earth shattering if you don't. I care more deeply about those who are close to me. I'm still a rubbish friend now and again and at times a dreadful mother and an inconsiderate neighbour, but my heart is now well and truly in the right place. And this has happened because of what I've been through. It's made me a kinder person and this feels extraordinarily good. In this sense I've never been happier.

My point is this: if we could count on everybody being entirely well-intentioned then I think assisted dying would be a good thing. Every case would be judged so carefully on its own merits and nothing would be done that was not right and kind. Finding a one size fits all solution to illness and death cannot, in my humble opinion, be done. It will always be a bit messy and fundamentally unfair to many people. But if I had to come down on one side of the argument or the other (which gratefully I don't as I continue to dodge the issue) I think we do have it about as good as it can be at the moment. I don't think the law should change readily, I am convinced it should be difficult. The money issue is unfair; but I think that's a price we have to pay.

I hope I've made a contribution to the debate by telling our story. I hope that I continue to contribute by talking to others and mostly I hope that I add to a growing voice that wants us all – children included – to think more about death. To not be terrified of it coming, but to understand that it will come and because of that fact we must not waste a minute in living the best life we can.

***

I cannot in all honesty say Simon's death was anything but calm and dignified. Not everybody gets a death like his. I thought it was a good way for him to die. I'm just not sure what it left behind for the rest of us.

Grayson Perry references Simon's death in his book *The Descent of Man*. Examining how the denial of vulnerability in men can be so unhelpful he states:

'The belief that self-sufficiency is a central plank of manliness can be so deeply

held that it becomes a life or death issue. Vulnerability can seem such a terrible option that suicide is preferable. Simon Binner, who suffered from motor neurone disease, was the subject of Rowan Deacon's beautiful documentary A Time to Die: Simon's Choice. Several times in the film, as the disease progressively robs Simon of the power to speak, then to walk, Simon writes that the worst aspect of it was the humiliation, the unmanliness of it all and that he would rather die. This was a funny, super articulate, Oxbridge-educated man, yet he could not bear to be unmanned, to lose his independence.'

This is just one view of course and it suited Grayson to make this point as it aligned with the messages in his book. By sharing the deepest intimacy on a daily basis with my husband, I had the best view of where he was. Although do any of us really know what another human being is feeling? The end game of MND is undeniably awful. But I think that Grayson is right. Simon's real terror was around vulnerability and that makes me feel uneasy. Do we as a society insist in a man not being vulnerable? Is it a generational thing? I do hope that the young men in my grandson's generation become more comfortable with this lovely, valuable emotion. Isn't it something that can bring us all so much closer to each other...

Through running our care company, we see these kinds of illnesses on a daily basis. I know how wretched these illnesses can be; driving families to absolute despair and exhaustion. But I've also seen how really good, kind, compassionate care from another human being can make all the difference. My family's motto is 'I see you.' The people we care for do not want to be viewed as patient A with X illnesses. They want to be Mr Jones who was a watch maker and a dapper dresser. He may have dementia but he won't wear a horrible NHS alarm around his neck in case he falls. It isn't sensible, but it ruins the cut of his suit. We help his family source a trendy alarm watch which does the same thing, but looks so smart.

When we broadcast Simon's film, a national newspaper reviewer described me as blinding myself with a false optimism that my husband could have a good, happy death. He said that I was fooling myself and minimising the dreadfulness of my husband's situation. I was bouncing along with false optimism that Simon could have a death like my daughter's. Soft, gentle, supported.

Well Mr newspaper columnist didn't know anything. I was doing nothing of the sort. I'd sat with the doctors when they explained the progress of the disease. I'd read and read and read. I knew exactly what was coming and it wasn't pretty. Death, when somebody hasn't finished with their life, isn't pretty however you look it. It's cold, bleak and unfair. The problem was I didn't want him to die. Full stop. Just like I didn't want my daughter to die. Every moment of life felt precious and that seemed to matter. Assisted dying does make grieving more complicated somehow. And that was an important conversation that we had with the doctors. They warned it would be harder for all of us; and it has been. Journalists! Honestly. Having opinions on things they know nothing about.

I fight hard for my optimism and I'm hugely grateful that I tend to have a glass half full mentality. But this journalist's comment seemed to me so naive and ill-informed. I suspected that this said much more about him than anybody else. Good health is such a blessing, but all of us will lose it to varying degrees throughout our lives. What I have found is that life doesn't stop dead if disability descends and that the flexibility and adaptability of a human being is a wondrous thing.

When my daughter lay dying, I sat with her in my arms, stroking her little head with tiny tufts of hair. She told me she was happy. Unbelievably, for that moment, I was happy too. There was nothing else of interest to me but my little girl's happiness and contentment. Our house was our sanctuary and it was a beautiful place to be.

This may seem the strangest thing to say but it was the worst of times and the best of times...I touched on love at its very deepest level. We think we are close to our children, but nothing came near that closeness and love that my daughter and I had at that moment. It was a precious moment and in my happier days it sustains me. I loved and was loved so much. And that is worthwhile.

In contrast, Simon's death feels unresolved. To me and I only speak as to bear witness, it felt angry, rejecting and abrupt. It felt a lot like a suicide. Simon was brave. It was incredibly important to him to be brave; to be seen to be brave. I think he genuinely thought that taking his life was brave and it would save us a lot of heartache in seeing him spiral into full disability. I know that his intentions were entirely pure. But I really think the words bravery and courage should be taken out of the whole equation. Surely it is equally brave to live with an illness, a disability, to embrace vulnerability and to accept that none of us really have that much control.

***

Death will come to all of us that is for sure. Why ever do we not explore it more before we are caught in its headlights. I'm with the Buddhists on this one. I've meditated for many years and follow the instruction to contemplate my own death every day. The one thing about losing a child is that my own death holds no fear. What I fear most is not living the life I have left in the best, most purposeful, way possible. I don't want to waste a single minute. I somehow feel that this is the best way to honour Chloë most of all. She's missed so much life.

I am more than happy to step back and allow others to make the difficult decisions. In the meantime I will go on sharing my personal story and hope that this in some way feeds into this extremely important debate.

*****

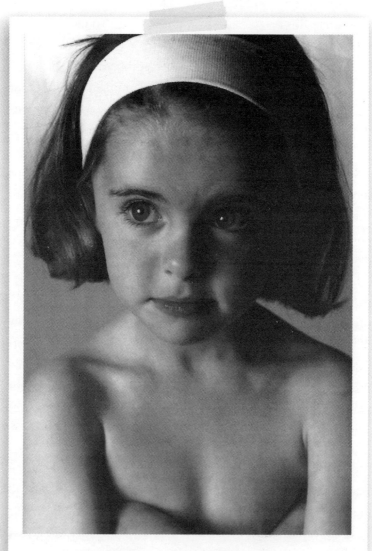

Chloë, my beautiful girl

FOUR

> *'I remember a girl so bold and so bright*
> *Loose-limbed and laughing and brazen and bare.'*
> - Nick Cave

CHLOË, SUCH A BEAUTIFUL NAME

AH, Nick Cave. He gets it. All of it. He lost his 15 year-old son who fell from a cliff near their home in Brighton. His son died whilst he was making his album *Skeleton Tree*. I have listened and bathed in his words hundreds and hundreds of times. They feel like velvet. So soft. In a first listen review, Jess Denham of *The Independent* wrote that Cave's 'experience of bereavement is blisteringly undiluted' and called *Skeleton Tree*, 'a beautiful, shatteringly visceral portrait of grief.'

My 18 year-old daughter's funeral. March 2013. It was snowing heavily. The church was packed. I'd been pulling these words together for a year. My subconscious, at least, knew that I would need them.

"Thanks for coming! How Chloë would have adored this! All this love and all these people gathered together just for her. Chloë loved the stage and here she is, right at the centre of it.

She'll be looking down on us and saying, 'Oh, no, Hannah it's Mum! She's so attention seeking. She's so embarrassing. Mum will use that awful posh telephone voice, and she's bound to cry and say something totally lame about me. Hannah, please stop her!'

Yes, Chloë sure liked to keep us oldies in check and delighted in telling me and Simon exactly where it was that we were going wrong.

How we miss that.

So, firstly, I apologise to both of my daughters that my eulogy will probably do all of the above. It will also be woefully inadequate in capturing the spirit of my beautiful, feisty and amazing young daughter. But I promise that, despite the most savage and intense grief, I will focus upon Chloë's life. A short life that, thank God, was exceptionally well lived.

Born 25th January 1995, she shot into the world determined to make her presence felt. She was a noisy baby, a tantrum-filled toddler and sometimes a nightmare little girl. In short, she was bursting with life, vitality and passion. She was argumentative, exasperating and totally adorable. Chloë, Hannah and I were joined in a vice-like bond from the very beginning. We absolutely adored each other and, of course, still do.

Chloë's beauty, charm and independent spirit meant that I was wrapped around her little finger from the very beginning - as were so many others - and she exploited it dreadfully. She just had a way about her.

I'm sorry Mr Hordley, I know that I ought to have helped you to mould Chloë into a diligent student. She was undeniably bright and full of potential, but I wasn't much of a disciplinarian. I indulged both of my daughters from the start, but I hope it was that blanket of love and certainty that helped give Chloë the spirit, the resilience and the courage to carry on living - and really living in a quite spectacular way - for the three years of her illness. Deep down she probably knew that her lifespan was limited, but in her words "Why go there?"

By 15, Chloë had blossomed into a beautiful young woman - leggy, with dark tumbling curls and huge greeny blue eyes. The world was at her feet; but little did we know that all hell was breaking loose inside her body. In February 2010 Chloë was diagnosed with Ewing's sarcoma, a rare and aggressive form of bone cancer that tends to affect tall adolescent boys and slim willowy girls. The horrible irony is that her sought-after body shape, made her susceptible to Ewing's sarcoma. We were brought down by a chance in a million; a Lottery win in reverse. There is no reason for this illness, no genetic links - just pure bad luck.

So how did she respond? Typically, she told me to 'man up' as she set about identifying all the 'hot boys' on the cancer ward. And there were many beautiful boys, two of them I'm so happy to say are here today. Strangely, we had some good times on that ward and bonded as part of an exclusive club, yet a club that no sane person would willingly apply to join.

There were some very dark times to come and I'd be lying if I said we didn't at times drift into despair. But Chloë would always bounce back and quickly came to deal with her treatments in the same breezy, cheerful manner - planning them carefully around drama lessons, parties and the commandeering of Hannah's ID card to facilitate Chloë's illegal entry into SHOOSH nightclub in Croydon. Sterile surgical gloves that the NHS funded to assist Chloë's cancer treatments, were instead used for fake tan applications. In full make-up and looking totally wonderful, Chloë would stick her arm out as the nurses pumped blood out or more medicines in. She didn't do pain, she wasn't squeamish and the nurses would have barely removed the last needle from her arm and she'd be up and off out with her friends into Croydon until three or four in the morning. Literally nothing would stop her.

I am so proud of that spirit.

I can barely hold back my tears when I think of how her dearest friends surrounded her with a cloak of love, fun and comfort. When Chloë was too ill to go out they'd all stay in with her; when Chloë was better, off out they all went. Quite a big deal for girls of 15 and 16 when the world is so irresistibly exciting.

Chloë packed a lifetime of fun into those three years, because she had such good friends. You were so young, you *are* so young, but you dealt with a very poorly friend with a maturity way beyond your years. I suspect you all saw me as a 'soft touch' as my eyes would light up as much as yours as I saw the beauty of you all heading off somewhere great and exciting. I think I got as much out of watching this as you did going. Lifts, the odd drink, opening the front door at six in the morning. No problem. They were some of my happiest times watching my daughter have such fun, with such wonderful young people, and knowing that it all probably wouldn't last. There was a real intensity for me in those moments - I really can't thank all her friends enough.

On Mother's Day just gone, that fell just a few days after Chloë's death, Sarah, Olivia, Rosie and Sophia sent me a card from my 'adopted daughters.' I broke down in tears upon opening this card. I've done a lot of crying over the past few months but that card really got to me.

I so miss the way you filled our house with the vitality of your young lives. I have no worries that you'll be back to tell us about your fantastic careers, boyfriends and, of course, you know how much I love babies. Chloë was just too important to us all and we all shared some really intense memories. I hope that in time these memories hurt less and inspire more.

Chloë didn't see her dearest friends in the last few weeks of her life; that was only because she wanted you to remember her with a big smile, high heels and a far too short skirt. The Chloë you and we all loved. She spent her final days with me, Hannah, Roman, Simon and Ralph. She gave us many gifts in those last few precious days - including telling me that I looked 10 years younger - very unlike Chloë and so I suspect that 'the morphine was speaking' when she said that. Chloë didn't do cancer and didn't do depression either. As we neared the end we snuggled up in her room and watched those dreadful *Housewives of Orange County* programmes and wonderful Mike Leigh films. She was poorly at times, but not that often. We ate fish and chips, still applied makeup and fake tan, laughed lots and little Roman would be bouncing around in the middle of it all.

Zoe, we knew you were there with us in Germany and there was a huge comfort in knowing that we could have called you anytime and you would come. Rosemary and Chloë Ridgeway you were there with us every step of the way and Chloë knew that you loved her so much - you were like an extra mum and an extra sister. Jacob (my ex-partner's son), your sister loved you very much and she knew how much you wanted to see her. She just couldn't but she did know.

Chloë's spirit in the face of such adversity was startling and amazing. My daughter taught me to seize and live every minute - don't sweat the small stuff and accept when you can't change things. She really is my inspiration. She took herself off Facebook when she couldn't join in anymore and then buried herself right in the love of her family. And how we loved that. It was a privilege to care for her and she showed such skill in protecting herself from emotional harm. Amazingly, most days she was happy; despite everything.

Some of Chloë's treatment was horrific and involved long painful stays in hospital. But she still managed to put cancer 'in a small box in the corner of her mind.' She'd be horrified if I ever suggested that she go on a trip with other children with cancer but would occasionally 'play the cancer card' when the benefits were too obvious to resist:

- like emotionally blackmailing us into buying her a puppy - we lost that fight pretty quickly
- getting to meet Prince William and to advise Catherine on false eyelash application methods
- and persuading me to let her go out clubbing the night before her Science GCSE exam! Oops! I forgot to tell Simon about that one!! Never mind!

Chloë died as she lived - complaining little and trying to see the positive in the reduced landscape of her life.

I've lost my best friend and half of my hopes and dreams (Hannah you have the other half). My family and I will never get over this - we don't want to get over it. Our challenge is to accept her death into the narrative of our lives without destroying anything else with our grief.

But at the same time, our story has been so life-affirming and we have been surrounded by the most wonderful love and support from a huge range of friends and family. You have held me up when I had no defences left and I know that you will continue to do so. There are far too many to thank here and now; but you know who you are.

My husband Simon and my daughter Hannah have been absolute rocks. And baby Roman a ray of sunshine to us all. Hannah, we are so proud of the way you've looked after your sister and we are most especially sad that we couldn't save her for you. We did try very, very hard.

There is one person I do want to mention - David Thomas - who lost his son Daniel, a Classics scholar at Oxford, not long before Chloë died and to the same illness, Ewing's sarcoma. Despite this you have been a constant source of comfort to me - and sometimes a partner in crime as we fought the various ludicrous systems that prevented our children getting the right treatments at the right time. One doctor once remarked that our consultant had the worst of luck when he had a lawyer and a journalist joining forces against him. Oh well.

Chloë's care at the end of her life was amazingly well managed. The palliative care team at the Royal Marsden and our wonderful community nurses settled into our eccentric little world and we all seemed to have a jolly good time most of the time. Their support was so fantastic that even my emotionally stunted husband Simon finds it impossible to speak of them, even now, without starting to cry.

I read the other day that there are worse emotions to have to live with than sadness. However vast and deep that sadness might be, it can be uplifting, invigorating, strengthening and above all a powerful reminder of how much Chloë matters and always will. My family and I will work hard to ensure we turn our current debilitating grief over her loss into something positive and worthwhile.

Outside our home, the care offered for teenagers with a cancer like Chloë isn't good enough. Access to new treatments is sporadic and filled with many unnecessary obstacles. Chloë was treated on a seriously outdated protocol and this needs to change.

Chloë was my inspiration and I'm determined to do something good in her name.

Chloë once said to me, with a smile and with her usual searing honesty: 'Mum I've caused you so much trouble; I bet you wish I'd never been born.'

Nothing could be further from the truth.

If, before you were born, Chloë, I could have gone to Heaven, and seen all the beautiful souls, I still would have chosen you
If somebody would have warned me 'this soul will one day need extra care' I still would have chosen you
If they had said, 'this soul would make me question the depth of my faith' I still would have chosen you
If they would have told me 'this soul would make tears flow from my eyes, that would overflow a river', I still would have chosen you
If they would have told me ' Chloë's time here on earth would be short' I still would have chosen you -
From *I Still Would've Chosen You* by Terri Banish

So, to answer you…Yes, Chloë, you've certainly caused us lots of trouble. But just give me the chance and I'd do it all over again like a shot. I am absolutely honoured to be your mother and I love you with all my heart."

***

For a mother who has lost a child there is no word more beautiful than her child's name. Please friends, readers, all say it often and don't worry about hurting me. What hurts most is the feeling that the memory is fading back into the mists of time.

***

Chloë Jane Drury, how clearly I remember her birth." Hasn't she got big feet," the doctor laughed. She did. Even as a baby she was colt-like with long delicate limbs. So beautiful to gaze at, but holding within them the start of it all.

Huge blue, green eyes. Dark curls. Olive skin. Ah the beauty of the Irish. To me there is nothing like it. The dancing eyes, the delicate cheekbones and dark heavy eyebrows. I sang to her the song my mother would lull me to sleep with as a child, 'In Dublin's fair city where the girls are so pretty...'

My relationship with her father was already over. We were never meant to be and it was a relief really on both sides when it ended. My mother was long dead. My family, which had once been a big, warm, loud one, now scattered all around the world like little bits of wreckage. I felt entirely alone with this little child. Her elder sister Hannah wasn't quite four. But far from being unnerved by the thought I was filled with an extraordinary power. I was invincible and I would protect this little child with all of my might. The power of a mother's love. She would want for nothing, ever. I would give my life over to her and her sister. My children were, still are, everything to me. Nothing has ever come close to the pleasure of having had my girls.

I am continually haunted by the fact that I couldn't make my daughter live, that I didn't protect her. Magical thinking? Arrogance over my own powers again? Who knows. I get the intellectual argument. But a mother's love runs so deeply through the veins. I failed my daughter. I don't care what anybody says. I fought the fight of my life and I lost. This will be with me until the day I die. And I've made friends with it - it's the only way. Otherwise it would have destroyed me. I failed and I failed in the most spectacular way. My child died.

I completely understand why mothers - I'm limiting this to mothers as I haven't been a father - kill themselves after losing a child. I so want to tell people not to. But who am I to do that? One of the main challenges of losing a child is that you go on living. All I can say is that five years later I'm glad I didn't kill myself. What would this have done to my other daughter? But not just that – what a waste of life. For me it would have been the easy way out. Shutting down the pain yes, but at what cost and what a selfish thing it would have been.

And I like to think that I'm not selfish – few mothers are when it comes to their children – or one who takes the easy option. No, the remarkable thing to do is to live and to somehow live with the pain of the loss eating and corroding everything good. That is the real challenge.

***

I gazed around the maternity ward and was puzzled by all the hoards of families - aunties, uncles, grandparents, others. Like many times in my life before I was by myself. When a family fractures early, through my mother's death in my case, you expect the family to pull together to soothe and calm each other. Not in my case. Sometimes the pain is too much so the family scatters. And my family had scattered far, far away - a brother in Portugal, a much older sister in America. A poor relationship with the children's father meant we had few friends. I notice in life that people pull away from toxic relationships like they sense it just isn't right. I gaze back at the young woman I was in that bed with her beautiful baby and I feel sad for her. But at the time I felt I had won the jackpot. Another baby girl. We were now a family of three. And all girls! What fun we would have.

And we did. For 15 years we had a ball.

***

A full-on feisty girl - we make them like that in my family - Chloë burst into childhood with charm, good looks and was thoroughly spoilt. Loved by teachers and children and most people who met her, she seemed to glide through life in a haze of good feelings, popularity and a general sense that she was pretty blessed. She was the popular girl in the class. She had the world at her ballet shoe-clad feet; little did we know that all of the pain and heartbreak lurking close by, ready to shatter our happiness into a million tiny pieces

***

I'd been on my own for a while when Simon Binner came into my life. I was 36. Who said dreams can't come true at that age? We met at a dinner party. He was hugely annoying and I didn't fancy him at all. Didn't even cross my mind and he didn't mutter a word to me all night.

I later discovered this was actually his 'treat 'em mean, keep 'em keen' strategy. In truth, by not speaking to me it meant I had no impression of him at all. He could have saved himself a lot of bother and just let me know who he was because he turned out to be really quite wonderful.

It was very strange when a week later Simon called me and asked me out to dinner. I really wasn't sure I wanted to go. I'd just come out of a relationship and was quite enjoying being on my own with my children. I agreed, out of politeness more than anything else. Later that week I cancelled. I just wasn't sure. But Simon was always patient and very used to plotting a path to get what he wanted. Eventually I agreed to go out with him and not to cancel.

It was a good date. He had a kind of boyish charm and, to my utter surprise and joy, a razor sharp wit. He was funny. So funny. Have I said that already? He had an enormous appetite for life. His intentions were clear from the off. He wanted a serious relationship and to get married. It took us six months. We got married in an old fashioned way. White dress, morning suit. There were blue and white flowers everywhere. It was elegant and it was dignified. It was the first time in my life that anything like that had happened to me. I always thought I was destined to need to work extraordinarily hard at everything and survive alone. It suddenly felt that life was giving me a break in the romantic stakes. I thought I was fated to always be on the wrong side of a relationship with totally unsuitable men. And yet here I was, blissfully married at last. Somebody successful, clever, talented wanted me to be their wife. I felt 10 feet high.

And things got better and better. For years I'd been a working single parent. It had been tough going but Simon transformed my life and gave me a wider family. His daughter Zoe from his first marriage immediately welcomed me and Hannah and Chloë and we were delighted she was now part of our family. I felt I belonged; we all did.

Simon gave me and my daughters, emotional, spiritual and financial stability. He was quite simply the most wonderful stepfather. He loved my children in a way I'd never expected. He put them and me first alongside his own daughter. It was a feeling like no other. It gave my girls security and a sense of being picked out for love.

I also want to pay tribute to Simon's family. His father John: super bright, loyal, strong, dependable and, of course, bloody difficult. A smart businessman, John was so impressive and I can imagine was a hard act for Simon to follow. We all adored him.

Jean, Simon's mother. Well another strong minded red-head, we clashed continuously and fought regularly over Simon's attentions. She drove me crazy but you know what, she gave me the relationship I'd been denied with the death of my mother. She never forgot – forgets - my birthday and she became a strong maternal figure for me. We argued and I continually moaned that she'd spoilt Simon so much that he couldn't even boil an egg. But she gave me something so precious. A woman of a higher generation who I could look up to. It was something that had been missing in my own life for so long. She made me feel a valuable part of something. I cannot over estimate how important that was for a young-ish woman with so little emotional support.

She was and still is funny too. It's where her son's razor sharp wit comes from. Extremely intelligent, she is full of energy, warmth and provocation. "Don't call me sweet," she said the other day. "Sweet means you don't have any opinions!" Well she certainly does have those - many of them.

Our house grew to be stuffed with even more energy, love, warmth and people. People of all ages. From parents to the girls' numerous friends. I discovered that far from being quiet and shy I had a hugely sociable side to my character and loved the house full of chatter and fun. Simon was strict too. A Cambridge education was a prized possession and he was determined my girls and Zoe wouldn't waste their natural intellects on too much TV.

***

By adolescence the boys started coming thick and fast. My girls were beauties. They took my breath away. I dreamed of the grandmother I would become. Of sitting back gently as my daughters took the reins and delighted me with all their adventures. I was on a real roll. Life was good.

And then the darkness came in again…and this time with a force I could never have really imagined.

> *'They told us our gods would outlive us*
> *They told us our dreams would outlive us*
> *They told us our gods would outlive us*
> *But they lied.'*
> - Nick Cave, *Distant Sky*

"I have a pain in my leg Mummy." Chloë didn't seem overly

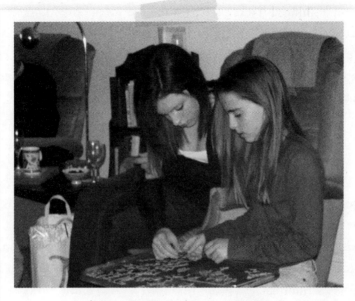

My girls Hannah and Chloë
– loving sisters

worried. Growing pains? A pulled muscle - she was a dancer after all? Let's leave it and see what happens.

***

Life went on. As a journalist and a PR consultant my dream job had been to work in international development. I was especially keen on working on something in healthcare with children. I got the job: Head of Communications for the Policy and Research Division of the Department for International Development. Quite a mouthful! I was ecstatic. I'd worked in fashion journalism, TV presenting and tabloid newspapers. It had been enormous fun but something had always been missing. I'd enjoyed investigative journalism because of the purpose and sense of justice that it gave. But international development offered everything – a chance to really care and that opportunity to really make a difference. Development ticked all my boxes; intellectually stretching, fascinating and important. Now, finally, I felt I had a proper grown up job.

***

"Mummy, my leg hurts..." Two weeks later her leg is still hurting. But I have that presentation to finish. I'll give her some pain killers, it will be fine. Don't really have time to visit the doctor and it's only a leg. Like so many parents I struggled with childcare for so long, now I was just getting a little more time back for myself. I was so fixated on my work I hardly heard my little girl's cries and I will never, ever forgive myself for that.

On we went again. It was October 2012. Chloë, aged 15, was off out with her friends. She'd started to go to restaurants and cafes. Wistfully I recall the tall, slender young girl in the bright red dress. The prettiest girl I'd ever seen. She'd captured the best of mine and her father's features. I lived through my daughters at this time. Watching them dancing their way through life. Opportunities everywhere. I was so proud of what I'd produced. So in love with both of them.

***

One month later. "Mummy, my leg hurts. Can I miss PE today?" Unusual for Chloë. She loved anything sporty. But the pain vanished for a while, or so I thought. I hadn't twigged that she was gulping back pain killers and that this wasn't normal for a teenager. Ok let's go to the doctor.

"Growing pains probably," the GP, a middle aged woman, barely looked up. She took her blood pressure. It was sky high. She dismissed it as nerves. "But I don't feel nervous," Chloë protested.

Back home. Only this time things started to feel more sinister. The mum of one of Chloë's friends called: "I'm really worried about Chloë," her voice was hushed. "Her back is hurting and I've used my pregnancy TENS machine," she explained. There was something in her voice I didn't like. I felt a sudden wave of panic.

Onto the internet. Leg pain? Back pain? 'Arthritis,' Strain,' 'Growing pains' kept coming up. But then I saw it:

'Children with recurrent bone pain must be seen by a specialist. Especially if the pain is at night and if it doesn't go away.'

My legs buckled and I caught hold of the sideboard. I felt it deep in the pit of my stomach. The world was turning in a whole new direction and life as I knew it was about to end. And to end in the most horrible way imaginable.

Having worked for the NHS in communications and being an avid supporter I don't believe in suing the NHS for these kind of things. But in hindsight the three doctors who saw my daughter were at best lazy and at worst incompetent. The signs were there way before she was finally diagnosed yet they just didn't go that little bit deeper. I kept going back for Christ's sake. Why didn't they listen more carefully?

Jesus! My world stopped dead. This time our GP visit was not so pleasant. I insisted on immediate tests. They gave in but sent me to the wrong consultant. Another week went by. Unforgiveable. Eventually we got to the right man at Epsom General Hospital, the kind of doctor everybody needs and wants. Warm, compassionate and 'on it' immediately. He was Greek and had that lovely fatherly gaze. He reminded me of the dad in one of our favourite family films *My Big Fat Greek Wedding*. He was a father. I think he said he had a daughter. I don't remember it all so well. But I saw it in his eyes: sheer panic. I suspect he knew what was up from the moment we entered that office.

"Girls of 15 don't get sciatica," he told us carefully. Looking back, he was beginning the 'talk' leading us parents gently towards what he already knew. My precious daughter. My clever, beautiful, black-haired girl was seriously ill. No, it was more than that. She was dying. "Can it be treated? Is there any hope?"

I was looking down watching myself speak. I had total disassociation from my body. This can happen when somebody is under the most extreme stress.

"There's always hope."

And that was that. I had, of course, expected him to say well of course we are near London with some of the best hospitals in the world. She'll need some time off school and there will be a lot of treatment. Blah, blah, blah. But he said nothing else and we went home.

***

The tests came thick and fast as the NHS sprung into glorious action. Off we went to a hospital I'd never heard of - and dear reader, trust me, you never want to hear of it - Stanmore. Built during the First World War, it's a sprawling mass of a hospital with lots of long, draughty corridors, very ill young people and the whiff of decay and age. It's truly the most horrible place I've ever been.

Strangely it also has an enviable worldwide reputation as having some of the best clinicians in the world. I got that, but it felt dreadful. Well this is where Chloë had her scans before we were told to trundle up to University College London by Euston station. Living outside Croydon this was quite a trip with my daughter who could now barely walk, but couldn't sit either because of the pain.

Once there we sat for, what was to become very normal for us, around two and a half hours waiting for the consultant to see us. Later I understood why the wait. How can you hurry telling a parent that you needed to amputate their child's arm, leg, hind quarter or that they'd run out of treatment options? Quite tough in a 10-minute slot. Still the wait seemed inordinately cruel and by the time we walked into Room 13 (yep it really was room 13) to see Professor Jeremy Whelan my legs were giving way.

I glanced at my daughter's face and my heart broke for the first time. She was just a child. The world was supposed to be at her feet; little did she know what was to come.

"We have the results back." Professor Whelan peered up towards us. He seemed cold and austere (although later I changed my mind about this). He chose his words carefully. "I'm so sorry to tell you this but your daughter has a tumour. It's a huge tumour and it's in her pelvis. I think from the x-ray it's most likely to be Ewing's sarcoma, a type of primary bone cancer that is more common in boys than girls. It tends to strike between 12 and 20, with 15 being the peak age of incidences. It's most common in tall slim adolescents and we think it has something to do with the growth spurt at this age. The good news is this type of tumour responds to radiotherapy."

Oh and it's 'treatable.' I learnt later that there was a big difference between 'treatable' and 'curable.'

I could barely look into my little daughter's eyes. I was totally engulfed by the nastiest, most horrible guilt. I had promised to look after her and I had failed miserably. She had CANCER for God's sake. My children were so perfect. This didn't happen to me, to us. We had it all. There must be a mistake.

***

THE DOORS OF HELL

'Suppose it's all true, and you walk up to the pearly gates, and are confronted by God,' Byrne asked on his show The Meaning of Life. 'What will Stephen Fry say to him, her, or it?'

'I'd say, bone cancer in children? What's that about?' Fry replied.

I remember looking up at the sign above the door of the ward and seeing the words Teenage Cancer. Jesus, how had we ever got here? Every part of me shrieked "NO. NO. NO." Not her, not me, not us. Whatever are we doing here? The denial lasted quite a long time. Looking back, the human brain must have been finding ways to protect me from the full emotional onslaught of transcending from a 'normal' life into an entirely parallel one. A world where parents, more often than not mothers, would sit by their child's side for months on end as they watched their precious loved one be pricked and poked, pumped with drugs, many of which have been derived from mustard gas during the world wars. And that was just the start.

The first family we met was Scandinavian. Tall, beautiful, blonde. All of them. The daughter, Grace, lying in the bed with a big cheesy grin. These children! The cheerfulness, the bravery. "I promise God that I will never complain again. About anything. Ever."

We said "Hi" as Chloë climbed onto her bed. The family was so lovely, but the horror in their eyes was plain to see. We chatted breezily for a while and the dad explained that Grace had been treated successfully for a while, but very sadly the cancer had come back. She was to have more treatment. She looked about 20. I struggled to hear the news. How could this seemingly, completely normal family be speaking so calmly about this?

The dad caught my eye and gave me a look that I came to understand and see many times on the faces of many, many parents. It was a look that said "Be strong. You will need all the resources you have and much, much more to get through a second of this. It will be hell and you will get so low that you will question the very reason of your being here on this earth. You will go to places that you will never have imagined. You will see all the lightness and beauty of your love snuffed out. It will be complete and utter hell."

He didn't say any of this of course. But in hindsight I know that this was behind his eyes. And just maybe too he wanted to add: "But unbelievably you will get through. You will live on afterwards and you will get through in some shape or other."

And he would have been right on all counts. I remember then that he got up. I noticed how well dressed he was. And his wife. That kind of effortless style that Scandinavians exude. He smiled and said, "Just need to shut the curtain."

But he didn't shut the curtain completely. There was a tiny gap and in that gap I saw the covers pulled back as Grace's bottom shuffled to the side of the mattress. She had looked like an entirely normal young woman. Very pretty. The only difference was that she'd had her leg amputated right at the top. She caught my eye as if to say "Sorry. But this is what happens."

We were right at the beginning of our journey. Naive perhaps, but I had never ever thought that children ever had amputations. Not children that looked so like my own children. In hindsight how arrogant was I.

I went on to see many, many amputations. I still shudder with the horror of it all. Grace, who had had a recurrence of her cancer, died a few months later. I remember hearing about it as I sat with Chloë one night by her hospital bed. The nurses were talking about it. She'd had her leg amputated, but that wasn't enough. Those vicious cancer cells had already escaped, lurking in her body ready to surface again in their own time.

The absolute worst thing I ever saw was a young man who had a tumour growing from his throat up into his mouth. He couldn't breathe and was foaming at the mouth. His parents stood in utter terror as the scene unfolded. The nurses and doctors, many of them only in their 20s and 30s themselves, in a full war zone with cancer. This was certainly the sharp end.

The boy. I don't remember his name and that somehow feels disrespectful, but I will always remember him. He was so brave, so gallant, so young. He bore it all and he died anyway. He was 19 if I remember rightly.

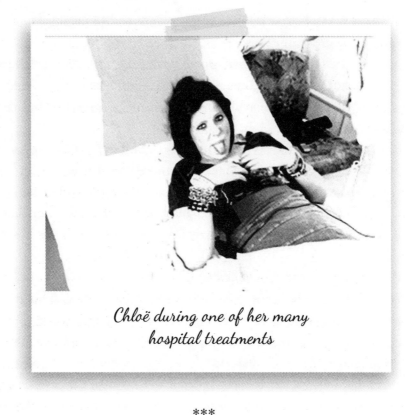

*Chloë during one of her many
hospital treatments*

***

Unbelievably there was fun too and we were of course dealing with teenagers here. Chloë, who had been quite a highly strung child in some ways until this point, decided to 'get on with it.' If I dared to shed a tear I'd be called out immediately. "Oh Mum, stop being such a wimp. There are children in here."

And never one to miss an opportunity she soon realised the dating potential of being one of the few girls on a ward made up mostly of gorgeous teenage boys. The fact that most of them had no hair didn't bother her a jot. And they became even more appealing when she had to shave her own hair off.

That was a dreadful day. Chemotherapy is described as a 'nuclear bomb' in the body. Sure it kills off the cancer but it kills off a hell of a lot else too. All fast growing cells are annihilated. Most significantly, although not most dangerously, is the loss of hair. All of it. Head hair, eyebrows and eyelashes. It is actually the loss of the hair around the eyes that transforms one from a person into a cancer patient. We just look really strange without eyebrows and eyelashes.

Chloë coped much better with her hair loss than I did. For me it was one of the most brutal transitions and a clear sign that we had crossed over into the twilight world of the sick child. In contrast she reacted with typical positivity as she quickly shunned the NHS variety of wig and found a luxurious real hair piece. At £450 a shot this wig was not within most people's budget. Even though I, like most mothers, would have sold the clothes on my back to give my child realistic looking hair. No need. In stepped surely one of the most wonderful charities in the world, The Little Princesses Trust. They fund the wigs and therefore allow the child to continue his or her life - yep there are wigs for boys too.

Wig sorted we had time to worry about the real problem of chemotherapy. Kids can take far higher doses than adults so the stuff they use is eye-wateringly toxic. It knocks the immune system flat and this leaves the body open to all kinds of vile and brutal infections. Anybody familiar with this world will know the drill. Chemotherapy for three days on a drip in hospital. Home we go and then five days later the blood counts fall through the floor. Taking the temperature here is critical. Any spike and we rushed off to the local children's hospital - in Croydon in our case - and put straight onto intravenous antibiotics.

Unlike UCLH, our local hospital was grim in the extreme. Mayday Hospital in Croydon. Nicknamed 'Maydie,' rebranded the Croydon University Hospital. The hospital is actually a really good one. But it suffers from the same ailments as the rest of the NHS, ie too many people living with complex problems, far higher demand and lack of funding.

The care was first class in every way. It was the crumbly old facilities and building that were so tough to take. So hard when you are in a side room in isolation for weeks on end in the middle of summer and you are 16 years old. The window looked out onto a brick wall.

The staff members were outstanding. Kind, attentive and knowledgeable and I continually reminded myself how children in other countries would not be able to access this kind of treatment. But boy it was hard. I've never seen anybody be so sick. Chloë had agonising mouth ulcers, shingles, extreme tummy upsets and was physically beaten to a pulp.

***

It is only looking back that I truly value the work of the Teenage Cancer Trust, the wonderful charity that works tirelessly to raise money for young people like Chloë and the many others like her. My beef with them was that they got huge funding and attention through brilliant marketing and great staff. But their focus is hospital wards, not investing in new treatments. A friend pointed out, "They can't do everything and what they do is really good." At the time I thought that they were wrong; now I think both are needed. Kids and teens benefit hugely by being in wards with their peers and allowed to have some kind of life geared towards them. And of course some – in fact most - children survive cancer so how and where they are treated is really important for their long-term mental health. But for those who don't, a cool ward seemed a kind of irrelevance.

I recall an occasion when Chloë had to have a tiny tumour removed from her lung at the brilliant Brompton Hospital in Chelsea. We had the finest treatment available but afterwards Chloë was left, aged 16, on a mixed ward! Many of the other patients were men and all around her was grown up talk about people dying of cancer. It was completely inappropriate for a girl who was really a child. With my pushy middle class pointy elbows I got her moved - but this wasn't really a solution was it? And this is what the Teenage Cancer Trust is all about - recognising that teenagers have unique needs. They aren't kids and they aren't adults.

What's more it was at the time, run by the wonderful, compassionate, talented Simon Davis, the most incredible human being ever. He campaigned with me to access certain treatments for Chloë. He was a rare breed, an executive who got his hands dirty, really cared and fought like mad for the good of teenagers with cancer. He was really brave too. Everybody loved Simon, kids included. I'm glad we've remained friends. He's since gone off to the States to run a US equivalent of the TCT. Our loss in the UK is definitely their gain. Whilst he was there pushing, campaigning, trying to do things differently I thought the organisation was really making a difference to families like mine. Really holding industry and others to account.

It is said that future doctors will look back on chemotherapy with the same disdain that our doctors view using leeches to cure people's ills. It is utterly barbaric and I remain so traumatised and distressed at the thought that I allowed this to happen to my little girl. But really I had no choice. We were told it was our only hope.

*****

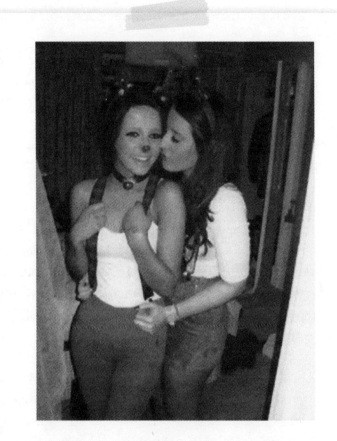

One of my favourite pictures of Chloë

FIVE

'Never doubt that a small group of thoughtful, committed citizens can change the world. Indeed, it is the only thing that ever has.'
– Margaret Mead

DISPATCHES FROM THE FRONTLINE OF TEEN CANCER

THERE is so much right about the way we treat children and teenagers with cancer. And there is so much wrong.

The distance of time has allowed me to look back through a calmer, more thoughtful lens. I feel duty bound to gather my experiences, examine them and then, if at all possible, use them in whatever small way I can to help other families. It is too late for me and my family but not for others who are already, so sadly, about to walk our path. Because one thing is for certain there will be others. Other families, other Chloës. Other lives torn to shreds by this dreadful illness.

Whatever else am I going to do with all that knowledge and experience? Using them to help others seems a better way of spending my life to honour Chloë. The best of daughters.

I was asked recently to speak to a group of new staff who were joining the palliative care team in Croydon in south London. It was the team that had helped look after Chloë. They said they were so keen to learn from the parents about how they could improve their service. I found it interesting, and perhaps not surprising, that it was this team that asked. I've found throughout my career that it is the team that does things best that are always looking to learn and to improve. It would have been a struggle finding one thing that could have been better in the way the team members treated us. They were without question outstanding. Their ethos of working alongside us, of considering the whole person, the whole family, of treating us like individual human beings made our personal hell – the end of Chloë's life – that tiny bit more tolerable.

The doctors, nurses and other health care professionals who we met during Chloë's 'journey' – ouch I hate that word – were almost without exception people 'on the side of the angels.' First class professionals who were doing a sterling job in the most challenging circumstances. On so many occasions throughout Chloë's illness I thought the one thing that was missing was that ability to step into somebody else's shoes and consider how it would feel. There were a few who did this brilliantly and it made such a difference. It made us – or me at least – feel less frightened, less alone, more like a human being and less like a patient. I think it's really important and something that has a huge impact on the quality of patient care whilst costing little or nothing at all.

So here are some of my findings from the frontline of caring for a teenager with cancer. To mitigate against comments of 'who does she think she is' I want to give some context. I was a mother on the edge, disagreeable, furious, unreasonable, demanding and at times driven to insanity through the pain of loss and grief. I was not the easiest of people to deal with...so my thoughts below are not intended as a criticism – we all could have done things better – merely reflections on the impacts of various parts of the system.

***

Today's doctors are adamant that children suffer more if they aren't told the truth about exactly what their chances are of surviving an illness like cancer. They point to extensive research that shows a negative impact on children when they feel that they aren't being given a full picture. They are most adversely affected if they think that somebody is lying to them or withholding information.

I accept the evidence base of this behaviour. But as I have thought time and again it's a bit more complicated than that. And in this case such an assumption can cause real harm and unnecessary bad feeling. We all have different ways of accepting information and communicating with our loved ones. Arrogant maybe or even misguided, but I do believe that I was the best person to know how to communicate with my daughter. Or perhaps even more importantly my daughter was an assertive communicator. She was making it clear she didn't want a full-on disclosure; she preferred to take on information in little bite-sized portions and even admitted once she preferred her information "sugar coated by my mum." Often she would refuse to come in to see the consultant. I thought that this was fine and allowed her a clear path to communicate through her actions in exactly the way she wanted to do so.

The doctors didn't agree. Some in particular were almost evangelical about ensuring that they bypassed the parent and spoke directly to the child at all times. Later I learned that they were concerned that the child was driven by a need to protect the parent, so as the theory goes, the child would be unable to ask things they wanted to because they were terrified of the parent breaking down.

My daughter was a tough little thing. I'd brought both my girls up to speak their minds. Chloë rarely held back in making sure I knew exactly what she wanted and that she was the important one. Quite right too. I don't believe that she felt she had to protect me. I think she knew that she had to protect herself. And she was saying loud and clear, "There's only so much I can take in. Be gentle with me."

For me the result of this 'tell no lie' policy felt at times brutal and almost verging on cruel. We never made any suggestions that we believed in fairies, dreams that would come true, bizarre untested treatments that were miraculously going to work, but I feel from the way that we were treated that they were terrified that we may go down this path. Maybe others had before? And by the way good on them if they did as in my humble opinion it is living without any hope that is the most intolerable of all.

I met some families who were clear that they accepted that their child was going to die. I met young men and women who had come to terms with that and who were planning their own funerals. I was full of admiration for their strength and ability to accept their fate.

But this was not for us. It was not for Chloë. My daughter, like me, was a creative, a bit of a dreamer. She loved talking about, planning for her future. The glorious future that she would have. We'd spend hours discussing her hopes to be an actress (no way!) a fashion journalist (better) and to live in New York. To buy designer shoes, sip cocktails. She would, of course, meet a tall dark American and live happily ever after. We had great fun with these fantasies and I don't care what anyone says, I believe that they were harmless and kept her engaged and happy. Even right towards the end of her life she wearily opened those beautiful blue, green eyes and said, "Can we go back to Corsica this year? I loved it there."

And I said: "Of course we can my darling. Of course."

***

I never told Chloë that she was going to die and she never asked. I believe firmly that she needed to hold onto hope and didn't want the brutality of that truth shoved in her face. I honestly think deep down she knew her fate and she knew that I knew that she knew. But that was enough; no need to spell it out. She found ways of communicating her needs. "If these latest drugs don't work, can I just stay at home?" she'd ask carefully. And I'd say, "Sure," and then gently shut the bathroom door and fall to my knees in total mental agony. Whenever did this world get so cruel?

I recall one doctor saying to me wearily and a tad disapprovingly, "Mrs Binner, we know how to treat these young people. We've been doing it for years. And yes I know how you feel. I've seen many, many parents in your position. You don't need to tell me how you feel."

This man was a lovely doctor but I sensed a frustration in this response. And if he hadn't been quite so lovely, I may well have given him a piece of my mind. Of course he'd seen various versions of my family time and again. We were nothing special. Just another family who were facing the most dismal odds and very likely to lose everything very soon. He'd looked into many faces like mine, faces who were begging him to just fling them the tiniest sliver of hope. And he knew very well that there was very little, if anything, that he could do. He was out of ideas and we were out of options.

I get how very difficult that is. Facing so many souls in pain. Day after day, year after year. All of them looking to him for that magic cure. And then blaming him, hating him even, because he didn't have it. Gosh the expectation must be such a burden to carry.

But he didn't know how I felt and I didn't want to feel like another hopeless soul. My daughter was the most special person in the world. To me. Just like the next child that comes in will be the most special to his or her family. I needed him to acknowledge that. Otherwise I felt he wasn't on our side and I don't think that that was true. I feared he was just shoving us down a conveyor belt full of the 'no hopers' and that he didn't care. And that felt very, very frightening as he was all we had.

I wanted him to ask about my daughter. Maybe even about me. How we ticked. How we got by. How we coped. How we got out of bed every morning for medical appointments - Chloë always ensuring that she was immaculately presented despite often vomiting before, during and after the car journey – and how we managed to drive three hours to the hospital and three hours home. All in the same day, every day, for months on end. I wanted him to ask how my daughter sat back and watched as her friends skipped through their lives with dreams of university, acting school and that whole big exciting world out there for the taking. How her friends were carefree while she had the weight of the world on her little shoulders. How I would cry myself to sleep each night, after my obligatory hours and hours searching on the internet for that illusive nugget of hope that would say 'try this and your daughter may live a little longer.' We were glass half full people. It's how we coped.

But that wasn't how our doctor operated. And as much as I think he is one of the most amazing men I've ever met, I believe that in this way he was very wrong. Of course he didn't want to peddle in false hope, but I think he – and may I say quite a few others – should listen more. 'Follow the patient,' that was the best advice I heard from Kings College London and the team there when Simon was ill with MND.

***

I'm still not sure how one tells a 17 year-old girl to forget all her hopes and dreams, to lie back and accept there ain't no future for you young lady. My Chloë had been ill for three long years at such a vital time in a young life. She'd missed so much school, so many rites of passage, from proms, to passing her driving test, to first boyfriends. She'd had a kind of arrested development. She looked like a woman, yet in so many ways she was just a child. It is generally accepted that such ill young people revert to a much younger age as they succumb to the need to be looked after.

Looking back I think the doctors knew from the moment we walked in the door that we had no chance. It's easy to tell really. It's the eye contact they don't make, the words they choose. Later they give it to you straight – the whole unvarnished terrible truth – there isn't any hope here I'm afraid. Move along. My daughter was my world and

I was a fierce, now furious, tiger mother. I wouldn't, couldn't accept this. I would not hear that my daughter was just another child with no options.

I literally spent every night, hours and hours, searching for new doctors, new treatments. Not in a million years would I accept their diagnosis. I fought them tooth and nail. All of them. As a journalist I knew how to work systems and boy did I work them. I got drugs other parents didn't know about. I'm sorry that they didn't get them too, everyone should get them, but I'm proud that I pushed open every door I could. A drug called Figitumumab had showed promise in Ewing's, but to everybody's horror had been dropped. The reason? It hadn't worked in the far more lucrative world of lung cancer - far more people you see. In short, children and teens get rare cancers and rare cancers don't represent ROI (Return on Investment) for pharmaceutical companies. Yep that really is the reason.

At some level I think I knew I was fighting a futile battle, but one look in my daughter's eyes and on I went. She didn't want to die. She'd had everything and then she had nothing. My life was meaningless next to hers. I've never been one to accept, "You can't" and this was the fight of my, our life.

Of course no world is perfect when you peer inside. And there are so many amazing things in how we treat children with terminal or life limiting illnesses. The doctors and nurses are almost without exception the finest human beings I've ever met. Nearly everybody is focused on a single principle of trying to help these kids.

But the system is battered – I don't believe that it's broken – but it is creaking at the seams...packed full of barriers, professional competitiveness which leads to vital information not being shared, extremely poor communication, silo mentalities and, perhaps most importantly, economic levers which mean that the industry cannot be interested in developing new drugs for children with cancer.

This really is a case for either governments to step in with some kind of moral compass, or private industry to put its money where its mouth is and make sure that commitments to social corporate responsibility actually lead to something. Or maybe even both. One thing is for sure there are new treatments coming down stream. Research doctors talk of us entering 'a golden era' of breakthrough research in the area of cancer. There is much talk of personalised treatments – that means one treatment for one person. Heavens this really is going to be expensive. How can we afford them? Do we want to afford them? Do our children matter to us enough? Of course I believe they do.

***

Children with cancer don't make money for drug companies. It's a simple fact. I guess we will all have to think more about how much a child's life is worth to us. As a society. Whilst I have breath in my body I will continue to try and raise the awareness of this issue. Fortunately there are some marvellous, brave, committed parents across Europe and beyond who also refuse to give up and accept that there is very little they can do. Their child has died or perhaps got better. Now are we really expected to go quiet and to shuffle off back to our old lives? Well it won't happen. We join forces with doctors, researchers and people in the pharmaceutical industry who want to make things better. There are some outstanding examples of people who want to do this. We talk, we shout, we attend meetings, we campaign, we make a nuisance of ourselves. We believe that there may be a time when no child dies of cancer. We know that that would be the best legacy for the children that we have lost.

We all get life so wrong sometimes don't we? Despite what I've been through I sometimes still say the daftest things to friends who are going through some horrible life stage. I chastise myself, "Debbie! Surely you of all people should know better." But what I have discovered is that most people, especially those working in the field

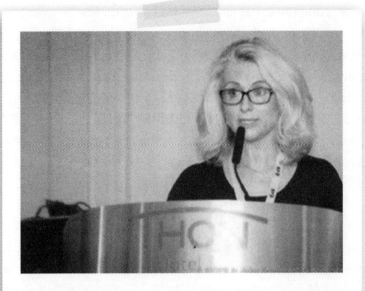

Campaigning in Brussels for better drugs for young cancer sufferers

of childhood cancer, desperately want to make things better. They are just human and need to find coping strategies like the rest of us. I just wonder if it might not be helpful to have less of an 'us and them' mentality in healthcare generally. I note more recently how UCLH in its amazing state of the art new cancer centre has done away with the doctor's desk. It struck me towards the end of Chloë's life how much better this felt. I sat alongside the consultant. Alongside, not opposing, such a tiny gesture that felt that something had shifted. It felt a hell of a lot better.

Another game changer was the back pack that allowed Chloë to have fluids pumped into her without staying in hospital. I want to bow down and honour whoever invented this simple contraption. Children HATE hospitals. Maybe we all do. The single most difficult part of Chloë's cancer was the days and days she had to spend in hospital. Much of that time was needed because patients having chemotherapy need to have lots and lots of fluids pumped into their bloodstreams too. This takes huge amounts of time and is one of the reasons that hospital stays are so long. Hey presto! Here's your backpack off you go. The length of hospital stays slashed in half. Just like that.

See there are some truly amazing things happening too. And that is just great to see.

It's over five years on now and I can barely bring myself to walk, or even drive, past University College London on the Euston Road. I dodge St Pancras whenever I can – too familiar to the journey to the hospital - and even Regent's Park is out. I'd often walk in those grounds with my daughter to see the trees, to breathe in the fresh air. To feel life again. Such a contrast to the cloying smell of the teenage cancer ward where all those drips were full of the most ghastly poison – the only option for so many of those children.

There are so many ghosts there. My daughter's little face as they hurled more bad news at her. Her wincing in pain as they passed another needle into another part of her young body.

My friend Rebecca and her son Eymen. A Turkish boy who was so handsome that he made me, Chloë and most of the women and girls on the ward, literally gasp in admiration. I held his mother as she collapsed in my arms after she heard that there was no treatment left after his third relapse of leukemia. I still well up when I think of that moment. I recall that, despite his bleak predicament, he carried on looking like a film star of a bygone age – chiseled jaw, flawless tawny skin and that twinkle in his eye. He died of his cancer. I don't remember how old he was. But he was very young.

That ward on floor 12 was a twilight zone indeed. It was where things happen that if there was, is, a God he or she needs to seriously step in now. How lives fell apart in a moment. Wailing came from the closed rooms – the ones where the most seriously ill children went –

and parents came out like zombies. The battle lost, the nightmare of living without their child about to commence.

So many children and young people died in that ward. All those poor families destroyed. And yet the fact that the Teenage Cancer Trust exists and runs that ward with the lightest touch is a miracle too. So much happens there that is joyous also. Popstars visit, there's a pool table, activities, a school; a little community that is full of hope. And despite my reservations about some of the practices, the kindness of the people who work in this field is so obvious and uplifting.

I noticed especially that the people who work in palliative care strangely, conversely maybe, appeared the most balanced, cheerful, joyful people I've ever met. I often wondered was it because they'd kind of made friends with dying. Hospitals are not great places for people who are about to depart this world. I've always thought that medicine wants to dispatch the terminally sick quickly as they are proof that medicine has its limits and can't make everybody better. The dying are a kind of living failure. But people in palliative care are different. I love the way they say that the real skill at this point is about working with families and allowing the child to live in whatever limited circumstances they have to deal with. Living here and now is key. Dying comes later.

I like this view.

***

WHY I CHOOSE TO CAMPAIGN

It's interesting to me that when I write about children's cancer, when I talk about it, present on it, fight about it I am hurled back to when my daughter was ill. But not in a bad way especially. I feel that fire, that passion, that need to make a difference. I see all of those children's faces, the ones that never got a chance to get better, and

I want to scream "We need to do better than this!" It moves me like nothing else.

I don't feel the same about assisted dying. This subject makes me feel uneasy, unsure of my ground. I would not be a good campaigner in this world as I just don't feel sure enough.

But children, that is a different matter. As I've touched on already it was a huge shock to me to learn early in Chloë's illness that far from being at the front of the queue when it came to ground breaking treatments, children were firmly at the back. I still find this shocking.

The reasons are, to be fair, complicated. I'm convinced the main block is that they don't make pharmaceutical companies rich. But there are other issues too. The rule of unintended consequences means that European regulations set up to protect children, actually cause a further disincentive to research new drugs for them. The pendulum has swung so far towards safety that experts now agree that the real challenge is how do we protect children from the lack of research.

Chloë was treated on a protocol that used drugs that were 30 to 40 years old. There was pretty good clinical evidence to show that the treatments, which involved four extremely nasty chemotherapy drugs, would almost definitely fail. What's that quote about the definition of madness is doing the same thing over and over again and expecting a different result...?

During Chloë's illness I had the pleasure to meet the extraordinary Lord Maurice Saatchi. I had long admired his work and although his politics are a long way away from mine, I agreed with the common thought that he was something of an advertising genius.

I first came into contact with him after Chloë had been refused access to a promising new drug trial because she was 17 and three quarters. Not 18. These were the rules so Chloë wasn't allowed onto the trial even though she was dying and there was nothing else to try. I know that clinical trials have to adhere to strict rules – somebody wrote to me to remind me of this fact. But I'm afraid this just simply isn't good enough. There was a drug, there was a dying child; it was available. She should have been allowed onto that trial. It was inhumane, unfair and caused our family even more pain and anguish when she was turned down. For Chloë it took away another bit of hope.

Anyhow my MP at the time Paul Burstow was sufficiently disturbed by this case to call a meeting at the House of Lords. Dear Simon Davies of the Teenage Cancer Trust, hosted the meeting. I presented and told the doctors and politicians there my story. There wasn't a person in the room who thought I didn't have a case. The trouble was there was a feeling of: 'Yes we know this is totally unfair, we want to do something, but we don't know what to do.'

Douglas Slatter, a former clerk of the House of Lords, a well-known gay rights activist, and one of the cleverest most insightful people I've ever met in my life, was at the meeting. He was policy adviser for Lord Saatchi who at the time was trying to push his Medical Innovation Bill through Parliament. Saatchi's wife Josephine had just died of ovarian cancer. Through her treatment he had seen, what so many others before him also had, that getting a rare disease is not a great idea as medical research does not see you as a priority. All down to that ROI thing again - not enough people, not enough drugs.

The Bill was really something of a Trojan horse. The great advertising man knew he needed a simple message to crack through the system. His message was around trying to loosen the legal restrictions on doctors prescribing off-label medication. That is medication that has not been approved to be used on a particular illness but where there is reasonable evidence to think it may work. This is really useful when people run out of options and are more willing to try something that throws them a possible lifeline.

***

I bonded with Douglas immediately. He was a whacky, exciting, interesting character. He was a natural disrupter. A natural campaigner. Through him I worked on the Saatchi initiative for a while, mainly around media and communications. I'd lunch with Douglas often at the Ivy Club in Soho. Sometimes he'd turn up in a stylish cream safari suit, on other occasions he'd be dressed in black leather from head to foot. He'd tell me: "The key to good campaigning is never to become like them. If they wear grey, wear pink. Stand out. Disrupt. Do something different and disrupt the system. It's the only way to get change."

Douglas died last year. I knew he'd been poorly – he was one of the longest survivors of an early diagnosis of HIV. I'd lost touch with him as the Medical Innovation Bill was taken over by the Government and became the Access to Medical Innovation Treatments (Innovation) Act 2016. But he sent me a message through a friend. I was beyond touched: "She was right what she was saying and nobody was listening. But she kept saying it and I think she will keep on saying it. And eventually they will listen because how we treat people with rarer illnesses is not right and it needs to change."

***

I think what I learnt from the Saatchi work is that change takes an extremely long time. A loud disrupter is good, but the real magic happens in the long run. The hard gruelling work of keeping on keeping on. Saying the same thing and refusing to back down or go away. I believe from the very bottom of my heart that we need a new model of drug development that brings in a moral lever. We need to accept that private industry cannot carry all the risk of drug development. We need a new way of all stakeholders working together around a common ethos that says our children deserve more than this.

I feel things are changing a tiny bit. And maybe as long as we keep on talking, joining forces with those people who want to make a difference

I think in the future things will be better for children like Chloë.

But there is much work to do. Today if a 15 year-old walked into a clinic with the same illness as Chloë she would have exactly the same chance of survival. That is virtually nil! And that is why I have now dedicated myself to work right in the centre of drug development as an advocate and a campaigner. I doubt I, or my fellow campaigners, will make much of a difference in our lifetime but just maybe we will help nudge the conversation in that direction. I really, really hope so.

***

THE BEAST – EWING'S SARCOMA

Two such awful words!

As I've already explained, Ewing's sarcoma is a form of primary bone cancer. Primary meaning that's where it starts. It is rare, affecting just 35 people in the UK a year. It is the second most common bone cancer, the first being osteosarcoma.

Experts have no idea why it happens. But there is some agreement that it is caused by a chromosome moving out of place after birth. There's probably something about the surge of hormones in adolescence that may trigger it. Tall, slim boys and girls seem to be most vulnerable to the illness. Again there's some thinking that the fast growing bones may hold a clue... Numbers have stayed steady over the years and it isn't thought to run in families.

For a lay person it's so surprising how little the experts do seem to know and how disinterested the doctors we dealt with at least, were in family histories. For example I seemed to be one of many parents in the ward who had a history of bowel cancer in the family. Anecdotal quite possibly. But there seems to be so little study into an illness that is quite clearly so horrendous and affects only our most precious members of the community – children and young people.

***

SIGNS AND SYMPTOMS OF EWING'S SARCOMA

Please remember that Ewing's sarcoma is extremely rare. But if any of the following apply, it is worth checking that all is well. And NEVER take no for an answer. If you as the parent are worried about your child it is the best indicator of all. You know your child best. Push for a first, second, third, hundredth opinion if necessary:

• A lump or swelling that doesn't go away
• Pain, especially at night, that doesn't go away
• A fast pulse without any obvious reason
• Raised blood pressure without any obvious reason
• General fatigue without any obvious reason

Of course all of these symptoms are far more likely to be down to something else, something far less sinister than bone cancer. But if you're worried, check. Many GPs have never seen a case of primary bone cancer and they don't know what to look out for. A dear friend and bereaved mother, who is also a GP, is running a marvellous campaign to encourage early diagnosis.

***

AND MY CHILD DIED ANYWAY

There's a leaflet that no parent should have to see: *Preparing for Your Child's Death*. We knew that Chloë was dying. I'd probably known from the first time I'd keyed metastasised Ewing's sarcoma into my web browser almost three years earlier. That was a terrible moment. But my mind just wouldn't accept it. Every sinew of my body screamed against it. The raging power of a mother. Useless in the face of childhood cancer, its ferocity had nowhere to go. Only denial enabled any kind of life possible. I get that one can endure the dying of a parent, a partner, a friend. One can walk alongside and treasure memories and maybe, just maybe then, the brutal facts need to be faced. But with a child!

The Hospital at Home team understood this. And I will never forget their wary gentleness as they tried to pick the right time to explain the important next steps. That they would literally be moving into our house, that a whole room would be filled up with oxygen tanks - looked more like a launderette - so that the tiny bit of lung that was still free of tumour could sustain her, and us, as she drifted towards the end of her life. And mine in many ways.

I was so tired. I gave up about a day before Chloë died. It struck me that I'd never given up for a minute, or a second before that moment. Three years of fighting, battling, hoping, praying, loving, caring … I'd do it all again in a second. But now I'd lost and I was resigned. In truth I now wanted it over. I was utterly terrified of how the end would play out. There is simply nothing more agonising than seeing your child in pain.

Her death is so very difficult to rethink. Over five years later and I feel sick to my stomach remembering. We were all there. Simon, Hannah, Roman, me and Ralph the dog. Of course. And three angels: the nurses from the Hospital at Home team.

I truly do not admire anybody more than those women who work with children at the end of their lives. Their dedication, kindness and total commitment will stay with me until the end of my days. That is a life well spent in my humble opinion.

Helen, that was her name. One of Chloë's favourite nurses. I was drifting in and out of consciousness. "Please let it stop, let it be over." I couldn't help it; I needed the pain to stop. Helen stroked Chloë's head all night. She followed a strict protocol of upping the morphine just to the level to ensure that her pain and discomfort were controlled. Whispering quietly in her ear all through the night.

Ah Helen I hope your life has been good. You so deserve a good life.

Unbeknown to me, some of Chloë's friends were sitting in the garden holding a candlelight vigil as she moved gently towards the dying of her light. The thought of that little scene: 18 year-old girls at the start of their adult life huddled together as the reality of how very cruel nature can be. Well it's almost too much to bear.

Young people are so totally extraordinary given the chance. It amazes me to this day that they were so utterly devoted to my daughter. But then my daughter was so very special. "Like attracts like," my mother used to say.

***

I think it was about 9am. I knew she'd gone before I even looked at her. A mother knows. I gasped and took her for that last time in my arms. The others came in and the silence entered the room. That soul leaving I guess. Three years of every emotion one could possibly imagine finally coming to rest. It had been one hell of a journey. But, still, and what a strange thing to think, I would have chosen exactly the same journey if it had meant I could have had all that time with my daughter. My perfect daughter. Would she have chosen the same fate? I've no idea. But I do know that she lived knowing nothing but love. And maybe that is something worth having. I hope so.

*****

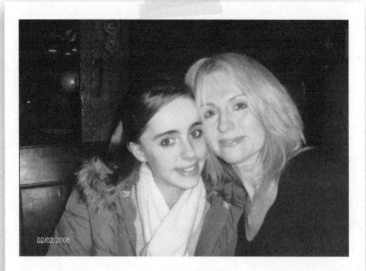

02/02/2008

With Chloë...

SIX

'I measure every grief I meet with narrow, probing eyes –
I wonder if it weighs like mine – or has an easier size.'
- Emily Dickinson

REFLECTIONS ON A LIFE

MY little granddaughter Nahla tells me "Nanny you are my heart." In her innocent view of the world she captures simply what we can all mean to each other. What love and family mean. At that point when we realise that all we really have is love and each other. To love someone so much they seep into the essence of who you are.

I am happy that I can love like that and summon that feeling in return. After everything, when my heart had been beaten to a pulp, it was miraculous that it somehow came back to life.

My daughters Hannah and Chloë were/are my essence. My life's work. It somehow feels important for me to leave footprints. A personal thing I guess.

When my daughter died I pleaded with people to tell me it would be alright. That it wouldn't always feel like that. That somehow, somewhere, sometime the pain would ease - even a tiny bit.

I wanted an answer from Sue Elfin, a woman who spends her days supporting children and parents with cancer, often terminal, at UCLH. Another one of those angels. A pure person who walks alongside us parents and families as we face something no one should never have to go through.

She is remarkable. Against the blackness, she stays sane. She stays kind.

But that day she let me down, or so I believed at the time. I begged her to tell me that things would get better. Jesus, I needed a lifeline. My body and soul were done. As a human being, as a mother I wanted it all over.

She met my gaze but would not give me the words I was so desperate to hear. "In my experience," she hesitated, "people never do get over this pain." Probably because she knew she couldn't lie to me and to have my trust meant more to her. I think she was wrong not to soften the message. I remember the room spinning and physically recoiling from her words. But of course, what she said was right.

That child of mine died five years ago. There is not a day that goes by when I am not floored by grief, but it is strange to say this but that really is ok. "Stay steady," I have learnt to whisper gently. "Just one step at a time." I am unashamed to admit to spending hours curled up in my wardrobe. Insane? Oh yes. Definitely.

But here's the thing. The light. The hope. It does come, I promise. Well it has for me and I was in a pretty bad way.

But I do believe that you have to work on it. Every day. And for me, the big reveal is that you have to embrace the pain. Sit with it. Try running and it will come after you and drag you back. And it will keep doing that until you stop and say "OK. I'm ready now. I'll sit and feel. Really feel." They say, "The only way out is through." I've found this to be true. It feels really horrible; but it feels better than running and if you keep on doing it then somehow it sits more comfortably and the jagged edges smooth a little. And one day it just feels a part of you. And that is a much better place.

'The pain of the loss equals the depth of the love.' I heard somebody say this once and it stayed with me. I've reached a point where I don't want the pain to go. If it fades so too would my memory of Chloë. And that would be truly terrible. My longing for my daughter keeps her alive for me. My pain is evidence that she lived and we loved each other so much. My daughter's name, Chloë, is the best sound in the world.

Everywhere I go I miss her. Everything I see I wish she could see too.

The best times are lying alone in my bed. Silent and still and no interruptions from the mad world. Just me and my memories. I used to lie in the bed we nursed her in, but not anymore as we sold that house. We lay in that bed, in that house for that last week. We lay there until she left this earth. I can still feel her long slender fingers in mine. Her perfect little face, so much more like a little child at the end of her life. How I held her up when she couldn't do it anymore. How her sister and I gently helped her to the bathroom. You really couldn't make up anything more tender. Pan out and you can see three women helpless, wiped out, but burning with love and a defiance in a silent pact to do whatever was needed. Hannah was barely out of childhood herself, but that spirit burned fiercely. She would not let us down. I keep that last bit just for us. But it wasn't horrible, or painful or stressful. It just was what it was.

We were beaten at the end but we accepted that. And in our acceptance we found some kind of peace. I'd had three years to get ready for this moment really. I had known from the beginning. I'd clocked the doctor's eyes, I'd read the literature. I knew. But to have told anybody would have felt disloyal to my daughter. So I never did. We never stopped fighting and we didn't give in but our hope turned to days, hours, minutes. How could we make right now better? A new DVD, fish and chips, a head massage. It was the ultimate living in the moment.

***

I hate giving advice to others about grief. How do I know anything? All I know is what my very personal losses have meant to me and how I have learnt to live with them. In my mind it is disrespectful to others to assume that I would know anything about their grief/your grief or how to make it feel better.

But I do know I have only been able to endure my suffering as I have welcomed it into my world and refuse to look away. Sure I've numbed it at times with everything, anything I can get my hands on, legally I should add. But gently and tenaciously I have kept nudging forward right into the heart of the grief.

***

GREEN SHOOTS

Education, literature and curiosity. That is partly what has saved me. Through these I have been able to escape the world and find a little space of comfort deep in my mind. My family has been central. My daughter, my grandchildren and the excellent relationship I have retained with my step-daughter and my late husband's family. And all of our dear friends. Be warned after deaths like these relationships fracture easily; it has all been too hard and we are just all too fragile. Misunderstandings loom and feelings are hurt so easily. How awful it would have been if those relationships had fractured after my husband's death. They are so precious to me. I tried to take care. And stepped gently. I instinctively seemed to know that this was the best thing to do. I'm really glad that I did this. Above all it was self-protective.

Another thing that has really helped is my love of yoga and physical exercise generally. A few years back, after Chloë but before Simon died, we were walking in the Dolomites in northern Italy. The mountains are my favourite place of all, having first discovered them at the age of 20 when I lived in a small mountain village in the Italian Alps called Ivrea. Peak experiences, those things that psychologists speak about. That feeling of being in the flow, of everything being aligned, so that you experience the most wonderful sensation of well-being. The first time I ever had that was gently skiing down a tree lined path in the Italian Alps just as the evening was closing in. If that is what heaven feels like then there is nothing to fear.

So strangely since my daughter left us I find them easier to access. I never would have dreamed that I could have found any peace or happiness after Chloë left us. The surprise has been the huge pain has allowed me to access a new level of well-being. It is difficult to take life for granted when one has seen so many young people never get to live theirs. How can one worry about getting old when my daughter and those other wonderful young souls, fought so hard to get that opportunity. There is most definitely a new landscape available afterwards.

Yoga too. It gives the mind a break, switches things off and allows a tiny drop of healing to take place. Slowly, slowly at first. But keep going, whatever your thing, it helps. It really does.

I am a proud à la carte Catholic. I renounce completely some of the harder teachings of the church and I've heard preached some shocking and unrepeatable things around abortion and HIV especially. And the church has been very unkind to me and my family at times in my life. Firstly when my mother was ill and trying to reach out. Secondly when as a single parent I needed a warm, kind place to go. The priest could not make eye contact and would literally throw holy water over me and offer me the chance to confess when I visited for support. My crime? – rather minor I hope you will agree - I was not married to my children's father. Now of course I find this totally ridiculous, but I was vulnerable and wanted acceptance at the time. I definitely wouldn't bother now.

My dear friend David, the grandson of a vicar, a devout Christian and a fellow bereaved parent, reminds me that I've actually been let down by the human interpretation of the church i.e. the priests BUT not by God. But whoever/whatever is God and where the hell has he/she been in my life? My views on religion are all rather messy. But then life is messy too isn't it.

I love standing in a church. I find the Catholic mass achingly beautiful. I enjoy my Catholic community and all my friends I have there. Two in particular have become close – Chris Rose and Sue

Nelligan – my friendship with them made even more special in that they were both my children's primary school teachers. These bonds run very deep. And they were some of the people who did scoop me up when Chloë died. How Nigel Bates, another parent and friend, seemed to appear as if by magic and take over the musical running of first Chloë's and then Simon's funerals. As a musician at the Royal Opera House, we were so blessed in having the most fine playset. And dear Nigel on the organ. It all felt so close, so intimate and my family were supported by this community in the best way possible. I guess in this way I was lifted up by the human interpretation of the church. I still, sometimes, wear a cross. When life gets really tough – my trip to Switzerland with Simon was right up there – I take my rosary and murmur the prayers to myself. Maybe it's the symbolism I like; a memory from childhood when things all seemed a little more straightforward.

***

Through yoga I have grown more interested in Buddhism and Hinduism. The mala beads, a string of beads used to keep the mind focused during meditation, remind me of the rosary, a string of knots or beads used to mark a series of prayers. Connecting with breath and focusing internally take me back to the calmness and serenity of the Catholic mass. So much criticism thrown at religion but what can be wrong with contemplating acceptance, thinking of others, being kind, not to be materialistic ... they all speak to my heart and give some kind of connection to other human beings.

I like religion. I hate division.

And yes I know I speak so often of connection, but I think it is this that is so very crucial in surviving - yes even thriving - after the blackness and stillness of deaths out of the order of things.

In researching my book I opened conversations with people who had inspired me across the years. Top of my list has to be Julia Samuel MBE, a psychotherapist and a friend of Princess Diana's, who wrote the ultimate bereavement book *Grief Works*. This book has everything you need to know about coping with grief. It sits by my bedside. I wish it had been out when my daughter first died. It would have helped.

She is a friend of a friend so I wrote to her and asked her three questions. Questions that I had been meditating on for some while. They were:

Is happiness attainable after the death of a child?

How does religion, or even other times such as the Victorian times when so many people lost children, help when somebody is grieving?

What about siblings and young friends? How do they fare when such a terrible event crashes into their young lives?

I am so humbled that she took the time to write back to me and here is what she said:

Is it possible to find happiness/normality again? There is no exact answer to this, obviously, because following the death of your child your whole relationship to yourself, your life and everyone in your life is turned upside down - but what people do talk about, following a long process of grieving, is that they find a new normal, a new way of viewing life, it is different to their past, but sometimes with the level of the pain comes an expansion of the self and an increased capacity to feel enriched by life - and their perspective of what matters in life changes too, much more about love and connection than success or material things. This can give them new experiences of happiness.

Can we learn from the Victorians? We can learn that external expressions of our loss, like black armbands, memorial jewelry, are significant markers which makes what is inchoate and invisible more visible and concrete. It means those around the bereaved person recognise they are grieving and may be kinder more sensitive as a result, people feel so lonely and invisible when they are bereaved. Both faith and the Victorian attitudes are helpful recognising the limits of our power as human beings, there is so much we don't know and can't control, and if we can accept that it can ease our internal battling and fury - all those 'what ifs' and wrestling with forces of nature they can never defeat.

Bereaved children. Children grieve by jumping in and out of puddles, so let them be sad bereaved children as well as normal happy children. Children learn to grieve by observing the adults around them, so if you show them your sadness and then get on and cook supper, or whatever, they learn they too can cry and then be ok too. The better the communication between children and their parents the better the family fare; they can often want to protect each other which can cause gaps of understanding. It is the quality of the parenting that predicts outcomes for bereaved children. With regard to children's friends, inform the form teacher or head, how to tell the children in their class about the death and what is unhelpful or helpful to say - our website has a whole schools section on this www.childbereavement.org.uk

***

GHOSTS OF THE PAST

Aren't we all unique; we all need to take care of assuming that what worked for me will help you too. I would often sit in the hospital alone with my daughter. Others would be surrounded by noisy, extended families and friends. I didn't mind being alone. In fact I never felt, or do feel, alone when I'm with my children. They were enough.

What did complicate my grief was my own tumultuous childhood. I was already well into middle age, but I'd yet to find those firmer footings. That emotional stability of adulthood that I now treasure so highly. When the world came crumbling down I was emotionally washed out to sea. All the footholds that I'd built up - a career, a happy home life, a husband - just couldn't withstand the ferocity of this life attack. They got swept away for a while at least and I was back in isolated terror. Worse, my little girl was looking to me to tell me it was alright. That it would be alright. Gosh I wasn't up to that task – at first anyhow.

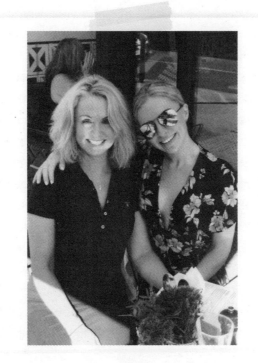

Me and Hannah

How many times have I wished that my early Catholic faith had remained strong. Personally I have never found a priest who has helped me. I've met some OK ones and some pretty horrendous ones. One particular gentleman stands out as getting drunk on my mother's sherry as she tried to seek solace from the church when dealing with my older sister who had a serious mental health issue (more about that later).

But this doesn't stop me going to church or having my own private deal with some kind of spirituality. I'm not sure I'm yet on speaking terms with God. Maybe one day. Having a church to visit, a candle to light, a sacrament to share – it has all helped.

***

Since Chloë died, and all through Simon's illness, I set about a program of self-discovery. I worked with a number of excellent therapists and health professionals. I believe that this has been another pillar in ensuring that I have survived in some shape and am now ready to play a useful part in the world again. Entirely personal, but I wanted to control my story. In order to do this I had to delve back into my rather bizarre childhood; to understand, to unpack all of the things that had happened and to put them back into their rightful place. I had had a challenging background and early on the wonderful therapist at UCLH had warned that this would make me vulnerable, to what is referred to as 'complicated grief.' At the time my focus was on being all I could for Chloë and for the rest of my family. So I set to work on understanding better how I tick and to make every effort to be as mentally healthy as possible.

As part of my commitment to candor and honesty I want to take you back with me to a strange childhood that I believe set up the foundations for both vulnerability and, perhaps more importantly, resilience.

***

I have two versions and as the old saying goes, 'the truth is probably somewhere in between.' The first is bathed in a pale yellow light - so reminiscent of those old photographs from the 1970s. I am standing by our apple tree in our lovely garden in Streatham, in south London. I'm holding our pet tortoise. I have red hair, wear a little spotted purple dress and I look so sweet and happy. While looking through old photographs, my children told me I looked like Orphan Annie. I can certainly see the resemblance.

There's something about red-headed children. We always feel slightly different, slightly off-centre. In a good way, I think. I don't have my red hair anymore. It faded and my love of glamour sent me blonde. I fit in better as a blonde woman.

We were 'well off' for the time. We lived in a nice street with lots of families and children - I'm still friends with some of those people now. Many of our neighbours were doctors, engineers and company directors. I guess we'd just made it into being the new middle class.

I was happy, sometimes, although I recall this was mainly when playing alone. Something I did often. I needed the solitude to recharge; I still do. I'm not sure that my friends would agree but I started off, and still feel, underneath, a sensitive soul. The challenge was my family didn't do sensitive and south London, especially at that time, demanded a more robust character just to survive.

I've always been good on the stage, so it wasn't too difficult to paint myself a different persona. I was often described as 'tough, spirited, ambitious.' Words that my parents seemed to approve of and characteristics that were most useful later in my jobs in a highly charged, male dominated industry – namely newspaper and TV newsrooms. I quickly found that by acting tough and brave it started to become part of my personality, or perhaps it was always lurking there. Whatever it was I knew early on that deep inside I had a huge pool of spirit and resilience to draw from. This doesn't mean I wasn't scared and very vulnerable at times, it's just I always knew I'd be ok in some way. I've seen this in other people and think it's hugely valuable. I have NEVER cried at work; but cried plenty of times behind a locked toilet door.

As a child, I was well fed, well dressed and well educated. We went to church every Sunday and I played happily with the children in the street. I had a bike and a full trophy cabinet of accolades in my two favourite sports: horse riding and ice skating. The house was packed with a menagerie of animals - a dog, a cat, a bunny rabbit, gerbils, budgies and various creepy insects. I have happy memories of the animals.

I was the youngest of three children. A brother three years older and a sister 13 years older. My parents were incredibly glamorous, good looking and fiercely intelligent. Being attractive, being successful, being the 'perfect' family meant a lot to them. My mother was an artist - in so many ways - with great taste. The house was kitted out like an early day Habitat with orange swirly wallpaper and purple duvets. We had Liberty print sofas and gorgeous, sumptuous curtains. Mother drove a red convertible Triumph Herald; Dad was chairman of the local Chamber of Commerce and ran a successful publishing company. My house was always fizzing with energy; not always in a good way.

But I must have been unhappy too. At 15 I was skipping my girls' private day school and hanging out with, what I mistakenly thought, was a far cooler crowd. It had a negative effect on my education. But worse in my parent's eyes, I put on weight. My perfect family did not do puppy fat. I recall the horror in my parents' eyes. "Watch the tyres of the car with all that weight," my dad's words sting me to this day. I tipped the scales at 9st 10lb – hardly obese yet I remember those numbers so exactly – but I felt like the fattest person in the world. Little wonder it started a horrible journey with bulimia. I guess it wasn't surprising really. I wasn't 'fat' for long – in fact most friends don't remember it as I'm quite a petite adult. But boy does that feeling and image burn brightly in my mind. It's like it overshadowed my whole teenage years.

What an utter waste of time!

Mother was from a huge, rumbustious immigrant family. My father had nobody. My mother was the youngest. She was a 'drop dead' beauty and always had the air of someone who expected to stop people in their tracks. For a little girl she was completely magical with her mink stole, mini-skirts, high heels and the gentle whiff of Chanel No.5.

Oh and gin.

And I still feel guilty talking about that, even though she is long dead. My mother was an extraordinary person, very much larger than life and funny too. The trouble was she also had a problem with drink. It started in a glamorous gin and tonic, martini cocktail kind of way. My multi-millionaire uncle Norman (a rough, tough Dubliner and former paratrooper, he'd made a fortune in demolition) had a bar in his house. Their family was so huge that they never needed friends for a party - it would be just family. I'm sure nowadays I would have found them great fun. As a child it was scary and there was a feeling of claustrophobia. Heavy drinking, belting out Irish pub favorites and then the inevitable fight between any number of my uncles. Things were always spilling over. Great fun, huge energy one minute, violent outbursts the next. To this day I feel nervous around drunk people.

When my family were sober they were enchanting. Not so much when they were drunk. And being drunk was just part of being Irish. Or so they said.

Meanwhile my dad would just join in. In huge contrast to my mother he'd been abandoned by his mother at birth. The story told was that she was a champion roller skater and had gone off to make her fortune. I've no idea if this is true but my daughters and I all ice skate well and it's a fun story that probably masks terrible pain. My grandfather was a stockbroker and by all accounts quite a gentleman. His death, aged around 40, was announced in the local paper as he was a 'local figure.' It said he'd died after a 'short illness.' Shorthand, I heard later, for suicide. My father always told me that he'd died from mustard gas poisoning after being in the First World War. My brother told me only four years ago that it was suicide. The stories we tell, eh.

Dad was hospitalised at 15 with TB. Throughout his life he couldn't get medical insurance as his lungs were so badly damaged. He went on to die at 96. Ha, the cards were on our family's side this time! But prior to that he hadn't known any love; he'd had to kick and push to even survive. He made a financial success of his life, but I don't think an emotional one. Maybe he was just a product of his generation; he had served as a sergeant in the Second World War. But he was an uncomfortable person to be around. He was volatile for sure. But it was more than that. It was as if he was looking for something and couldn't find it. He would look straight through me and I felt no love at all in either direction. The saddest thing is that I was hard wired early on to try and please him. Something gave me an expectation that I needed to make him happy. Little me! However, could I do that? But I tried and I failed. Over and over again. I was five years-old and remember to this day how I wanted to cover myself with an invisible cloak so as not to annoy him so much.

His temper was another thing altogether. It would kick off at the slightest thing. Our house continually teetered on the brink of his explosive rage.

He went on to live a long and healthy life. I've no idea if he was happy. He was incredibly sociable and had lots of friends. They would have said, I've no doubt, what a "great guy" he was. Fun, smart and a black belt in the martial art of Aikido. But he remained 'not present' for us. And this hurts me to this day.

***

'When I look back on my childhood I wonder how I survived at all. It was, of course, a miserable childhood: the happy childhood is hardly worth your while.'
- Frank McCourt, *Angela's Ashes*

When Dad lay dying - my Chloë was already ill - I kissed his cold head and tried to find some emotion inside of me. There was nothing. Duty yes. Sadness of course. Even compassion. But no love had ever passed between us and that is really damaging for a young woman and how awful for him. I wanted to love him.

***

When I reach back for childhood memories I feel a cauldron of emotions. My sister's mental illness casts the widest, deepest shadow. As I've said I won't go into it here in any detail. But this level of mental illness has terrible ramifications for the whole family. It makes home life feel scary and unsafe. The strangest thing is this feeling lingered with me until Chloë got ill. Only then did I truly get that life is scary and unsafe and at the end of the day there's very little any of us can do about that. That acceptance again; it was key in making life feel a tiny bit easier.

Whilst I was the perfect daughter inside of the house, I was very naughty outside. I was hugely attracted to danger, to anything exciting that allowed me to feel. It all culminated with me being expelled from school aged 16.

If only a therapist would have stepped in here things could have been so different. I hope from the bottom of my heart if there is any girl reading this and something resonates that she gets help now. Do not wait. Life is too short not to sort out the foundations first. Good parenting does it for you, but not everybody is that lucky. I wasn't, but I've subsequently done the work and boy does it feel good.

***

My mother was fundamentally a good person but it was the drink that ruined her. I thought everybody's mother had an empty bottle of gin under the sofa. But you never would have guessed it. She always looked immaculate and she had that Celtic charm that completely disarmed everybody she met. People loved my mother – it was a kind of gift that she had. I occasionally bump into people who knew her and their eyes light up when they talk about her. She was a very special person.

But her struggles with life, with my sister's mental illness, meant that she wasn't really available for me and my brother for much of my childhood. Keeping up appearances was vital to the survival of my family. There was such shame with mental illness in those days, it must have been agonising for my poor mother to keep everything firmly behind closed doors.

The result was I was left to bring myself up. And 15 year old girls are not the best judge of what is and what is not safe or sensible. Do we all look back and shudder at the risks we all took and marvel that we ever survived at all? But difficulties at home can lead to a kind of added recklessness. I remember having a strong sense of no real desire to live or die. In hindsight I think that was the beginning of a lurking low level depression. Although at the time I had neither the language nor the insight to identify this. I just thought that feeling sad was part of life.

I don't feel this anymore. I feel sad because of what I have lost. But I now have a real sense of what happiness can feel like too. I believe I've only been able to access this feeling because of all of the work I've done on myself. It's been incredibly hard, but so worth it.

In the dead of night I sometimes remember a feeling of terror in my house. That unsafe feeling again. But now I can rationalise and understand my parents just found life too difficult themselves. It wasn't anybody's fault; there just wasn't enough love to go around. Post war they'd had hard and frightening lives.

***

We humans often linger on the bad times. I must remind myself there were good times too. I'm certain that the more good times one can build in the mind the more the good feelings crowd out the bad.

America was a special place for us. At 55, having only ever been to Ireland, my bold mother decided that we were off to California . The America of the late 70s/early 80s. I was 15 years old and had suddenly discovered boys! It was so exciting. I got my first taste of Macdonald's, drive-in movies… We stayed on St Petersburg beach in Florida in the Hilton Hotel. (My mother was making her fortune in estate agency just as the property boom was getting into full swing.) I had a boyfriend who was a champion surfer. Life suddenly switched to good. It was so strange. My mother loved the States so much we headed off there, four summers in a row. Best of all, I had her all to myself. I lost the puppy fat that she had so disapproved of and was rather delighted to blossom into a beautiful young woman and found some self-worth. I loved my mother very, very much, in spite of it all. And this is the happiest of happy memories I have. I keep it locked tight inside me. A child and a young person need some hope. Don't we all…

***

Understanding my background has been important in my survival. To get the myths and the stories that are passed through the generations. To work out if they really help you. It's made me understand why I always wanted to please people and keep the peace. That I was obsessed with appearing perfect, slim and had terribly high and unrealistic expectations of life. If I put on a couple of pounds I would stay home and hide. If I had one spot on my face I'd even dodge going to work. I was only ever loveable if I was completely perfect. And as none of us are - I wasn't ever loveable.

Religion played its role too and the Catholic faith seems especially complicit and complicated in this respect. In the haze of my childhood memories I recall a terror at seeing a priest or a nun. They had 'superhuman powers' to see right through you. I remember the fear of first feeling sexually aroused. Guilt, shame. I swear I saw the priest - an elderly Irish gentleman who was as mad as a box of frogs - glaring down at me from the pulpit. He knew. I knew he knew.

The Catholic Church is great at evoking those emotions. Guilt being the main one of course. But since Chloë the tables have turned. I want the answers now. I said my prayers, I tried to be good, I obeyed the commandments – mostly - but something still let my little girl die. How can you tell me about a merciful God?

Yet I do not hold with those who ridicule religion as being nonsense and the root of all evils. I think it can be enormously helpful and can inspire people to do wonderful things. It's all in the interpretation. I'm envious, and respectful, of people who are religious – in a good way. I know some of them. They are stand out people.

***

MY MOTHER'S DEATH

And this is where it started. What Simon called my 'curse' – no malice there; just how he'd make things feel alright by making fun of them.

But first the good times. Back to America as it burns brightly in my memory bank. *Dallas, Falcon Crest, Dynasty*. My mother and I were glued to these programmes. And stepping off of the plane I thought we were stepping into a film set. A world of sizzle and possibility. I had a much older half-sister (on my dad's side from a very early relationship, long before Mum). Her name was Anne and she drove a Cadillac. Dad had her at 19, me at 50. She'd been an air stewardess when flying was really glamorous. She was married to Bob who was head of homicide for Los Angeles police force. He wore a Stetson, carried a gun in a holster, smoked Marlboro cigarettes and called me "honey." But that wasn't all. I had an uncle who was a film producer in Hollywood and an aunt who made Elizabeth Taylor's wigs.

We ate in a rooftop revolving restaurant in LA. We hung out with the most flamboyant fun crowd in Hollywood. I had earth shattering romances with Californian beach boys called Dan and Doug, made a best friend called Anne-Davey (now a well-known US attorney), we bought levis, baseball boots and I was offered my first puff of weed (I hated it for the record).

My uncle was gay, although my mother wouldn't accept it. She would say, "Don't worry about Uncle Denis, he just has lots of friends but is still looking for that right girl to marry." I think he was at least 40 years old at the time and I am very sure he was looking for no such thing. My mother couldn't help it. She was from a different age and a different time. Anyhow she didn't have an unkind bone in her body; she just needed the narrative to fit. Well Denis and his 'friend' were a hoot and made an unworldly English teenager and her lovely mother very happy indeed. We laughed, we drank. I thought life had started. I thought that this was the end of family misery and the start of something wonderful.

***

And then the storm. I noticed the feet first. My mother's feet. They were terribly swollen. Strange. But off we went; there was so much to do and the sun was shining. Today I was off on a boat trip with my new blonde, suntanned buddies. I thought little more about it.

On the plane home I glanced at her face and saw something. A panic, I think. Just a flash. Back home all hell let loose. Our family doctor – a lovely, kindly Polish man who'd been our GP since birth - whom my mother had stopped visiting some months back, appeared at the door. I remember his eyes. They were so blue. So sparkly. But was that a tear? I was confused.

"I'm afraid your mother is very ill." What? Whatever was he talking about? "She's been ignoring her symptoms but now she has a tumour the size of an orange protruding from her stomach." I'm not sure why he told me this. I guess things were different then.

Fast forward the numerous hospital tests. My mother was diagnosed with bowel cancer. She'd had it for months, maybe even years. But, later from her journals, I read that she'd tried to 'pray' it away. Well, that's what Irish Catholics did then. I hated the people that had allowed her to do this.

She had a massive operation at King's College Hospital, London. No chemotherapy. I think they knew then that the operation was about prolonging life, not a cure. I was studying journalism at The London College of Printing. My dream career and - later - to become my real saviour. Sitting in the class one day my lecturer called me over. His face looked grey. I knew what he was going to tell me. "My mother's dead isn't she?" I said, my cheeks burning with what I can only recall as fury. I felt my body tremble 'Don't show any fear, any emotion,' I heard my subconscious push through. 'You won't cope, it's too much. It isn't safe yet.'

"Good heavens. No," said the lecturer clearly shocked. "She's coming out of hospital and will see you at home." That journey home was the longest ever. I ran up the street. I wanted to see my mum. Feel her, check her, know that she was still alive.

It was such a shock though. I don't think I'd ever seen an ill person. Her face was sunken, her once piercing green eyes faded to a dull grey. She was so thin. Her glorious black hair, greying now and clinging to the side of her jaw. Where ever had my mother gone?

Miraculously she started to get better again. She went back to work. Bought a whole new work wardrobe with brand new high heels. She looked a million dollars again. She always had the most exquisite bone structure – I've seen the same shape in other Irish women. So off we went. I was a strange young woman. I had lots of friends who I liked very much. But Mum was my best friend. The room would light up when she walked in. Walking home from school my heart would skip a beat when I saw her red car parked outside. I never got to see her as an old woman. Not sure if that is good or bad really. I know for sure she would have hated it.

Mother got well enough for us to holiday again - just the two of us - in Italy this time. Mum and daughter back together. We stayed on the Adriatic coast visiting Positano, Sorrento, Amalfi. Bliss.

But she got ill again. Cancer. Darn cancer. She was sunbathing in the garden and I noticed the swelling on her side. I was so young, but I somehow knew what it was. The cancer had spread to the liver and she told me as I accompanied her to the consultant visit, "It's curtains for me."

I did the first shameful thing I'd ever done. I had never let my mother down. While a bit wild and badly behaved outside of the house, inside I was the perfect daughter. I knew I couldn't play up - even a little bit. My parents were too fragile and exhausted by my sister. There was no space for me. But this time, driven by a kind of self-preservation, I escaped to Italy. A country I had loved for years. I got a job working as an English teacher for Olivetti – its headquarters were based in a mountain village in the Alps called Ivrea - and left that day. I was about to combust. It was too much.

***

I wasn't home when my mother died. I was 20 years old. Instead I was with my lovely friend Alison, still one of my very best friends, in an Italian bar, sipping cappuccinos and gobbling down the tastiest brioches I've ever had. I was in complete denial. For the first time in my life, but not the last, I closed down completely from reality and developed a kind of alter ego. There was a strange feeling of disassociation, of stepping outside of myself. For a while it worked and it got me through.

But reality is always there. My boss, a kindly man called Graham, was waiting for me when I got back. I'd never especially taken to him, but this time he had tears in his eyes and showed nothing but tenderness and compassion for a young woman in pain. "Your mother," he said softly. People always surprise you don't they!

He didn't need to say more. The tears I'd been holding in for so very long erupted. My legs buckled and I crumpled. Devastated, defeated and so far from home.

That night there was an incredible storm. My new friends in Italy were so sweet and gentle. But I had that feeling of being picked out. There they all were enjoying their young lives and I wasn't allowed to. It sounds callous now, but it was my first feeling. I was furious with my mother for dying as sometimes that's the only way to survive. Mothers weren't supposed to die and leave their 'half cooked' children. Especially as she had now become the mother I'd always wanted. She was supposed to be invincible.

***

The sadness came later. Many years later. I really only stopped pining for my mother when Chloë got ill. This somehow put everything into perspective. I'm not sure that the 20 year-old mind can really take in the enormity of the loss. The absence of such a fundamental figure as one moves through the various stages of life: promotion, first house, first baby, marriage…

I feel so very sad when I hear about people losing a parent at this age. We expect them to be adults, so it isn't as bad as losing a parent as a child. But I think it is still really difficult. I don't know any 20 year-olds who are actually adults. It is a critical transition period and a guiding hand should be there.

Off I went, job on a local newspaper before landing 'the most glamorous job in the world' on a business fashion magazine called *Drapers Record*. This really was all my dreams come true. I'd found something I was really good at. Talking to people and then writing about it. Brilliant! Working in Swiss Cottage I was surrounded by interesting, arty, intelligent people. Loads of them. I went to fashion shows in Paris, Milan, Florence, wore all the latest clothes, had glamorous unsuitable boyfriends. Went to Ronnie Scotts, dined out with the media crew at Kettner's in Soho, got interested in Lorca the Spanish playwright. I grilled Harrods' boss Al Fayed on various retail issues, Terence Conran on the 'failure' of Habitat - he wasn't very pleased with this little upstart quizzing him - mixed with models, celebrities. I was flying so high. It was a fabulous time and I started to come alive. I'd found my passion. It was a golden, golden time and I'm so glad I lived this bit.

***

FAMILY LIFE

And then came Richard. My father didn't - no couldn't - love me, so no surprise I was instantly attracted to men who were either unavailable, cruel and dysfunctional and often all three. It was text book dysfunctional behaviour.

Richard was a fireman. I was in desperate need of a rescuer and there he was - on the surface at least. Tall and stunningly good looking. Fun too. We moved in together and had a couple of really nice years. Hannah came first. Red-headed like her mum, green-eyed like her dad. The sweetest little girl with perfect features and so very loving. I missed my mum when she was born. It was seven years since she'd died and I was 28 by then. But boy I felt her loss so much. It sounds so obvious but I was so aware of all the years that my mum was missing.

I have friends now in their early 50s who still have their mums. If only mine hadn't left so soon. If only we'd had more time to patch up the past wrongs, to become deeper friends and to really find each other. If only she'd met my daughters. Chloë, especially, looked so like her. But it wasn't to be and that still makes me sad.

Hannah was a delight and along came Chloë three and a half years later. By this time things had turned sour between me and Richard. In hindsight there is no blame, we were just terribly ill-suited on so many levels. I, fragile, hyper-sensitive with a deep sense of being unlovable. There was no way I wasn't going to walk into a dysfunctional relationship. I've long since given up wondering what he felt as it doesn't seem to matter anymore.

But the result was my second baby girl being born to a woman who was a little bit lost. No mother, no family, no partner who was really present. As soon as that baby fell into my arms I sobbed with relief. I knew I had to be alright for this little person. With both my children it was love at first sight. I had no issues just scooping them up and giving them my heart, my breath, my soul. My children really have been the love of my life and I feel so enormously blessed that I was able to have them - despite all that happened later.

At last, I felt. I can really do this and do it well.

My daughters gave me the chance to build a family again. To be happy. If only God had chosen to take something else from me. He really hit me at the very heart of my soul.

***

THE MIDDLE YEARS

As Chloë arrived, Richard bought himself a two-seater sports car. I actually find this mildly amusing now and accept it was a bit of a clue. There were many letdowns like this. Many a night where I sat alone weeping on the sofa as my two little angels slept soundly upstairs. I knew things were wrong, but I didn't know why and I couldn't find a way to make them feel better. More than anything it was just really confusing. In hindsight it was simply lack of experience and the fact that dominating men are very good at picking out vulnerable women and isolating them from anything that gives them strength. And in my case that also included my job, my work, the thing that has always given me the most pride and security in the world.

I felt I was nothing. There was no love anywhere.

***

Richard and I split up. I was sad at the time as I hadn't wanted that for my girls and I'd tried very hard to make things work. But looking back, this was a really good thing and allowed us both to grow in different directions. He turned out to be a good, reliable father and really what more could I ask.

For me it allowed me to get on with life, get out into the world and to really discover what I wanted to be. In the depths of something so challenging, I noticed this inner steel. Far from being a terrible time, it turned into a world of opportunities. I got back to work, this time as a TV presenter and journalist. I was driven on by necessity and a burning desire to make something of my life for my children first and foremost, but also for myself. It was first of many times when I realised that the best of me came out in what could have been the worst of circumstances.

The next few years were glorious. My beautiful children grew and blossomed. If only I'd realised at the time just how lucky I was. And then I met Simon and life really took on a new dimension.

*****

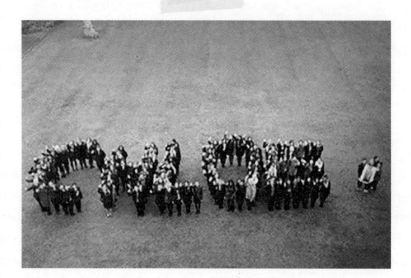

Chloë's amazing school friends.
I was so touched by this

SEVEN

'Would you rather love the more, and suffer the more; or love the less, and suffer the less? That is, I think, finally, the only real question.'
– Julian Barnes, *The Only Story*

CHLOË. SADNESS AND A SHIFTING LANDSCAPE

WHEN I first read Barnes's words I gasped aloud. You know that feeling when a writer captures exactly what you want to say in the most exquisite way – like the perfect piece of music. That feeling when that writer makes you feel less alone in the world. Like they're your best friend and they are speaking directly to you.

Those words shifted my perspective. I guess that's why I read so much; I want to keep shifting my perspective on life. It's hard to explain but I'll try. I think that this part is useful to you, dear reader, if you are looking for some comfort in your time of darkness. Or is that too bold an assumption for me to make? Your pain, like mine, will be unique. Anyhow this helped me. When Chloë first died, it ripped me apart to such a degree that I had nothing left inside. I felt entirely empty; both physically and mentally. I knew that I would never recover if I stayed in this place.

At first I got really busy. I campaigned day and night for what I still believe is the massive injustice that we live with on a daily basis; that is that research on children with cancer, and many other horrible life limiting and terminal illnesses, are not prioritised by drug research companies as they don't make money in our capitalist state. (That still makes me shudder with rage). When I wasn't doing that I was travelling, working. I was a human dynamo. I've never achieved so much. This was all interspersed by massive emotional crashes. Sobbing, wailing and the rest. But with me this was always firmly behind closed doors.

But the truth was I was simply terrified. If I stood still I thought the sadness would just engulf me. There was so much of it. I had to run, run, run. It was exhausting.

I've seen people live like this for years. In a no-man's land of utter despair. I've heard other bereaved parents say they can't look at other people's children, never do Christmas and their lives become shells of what was before. I understand this. But this route was not for me. I seemed to be mostly fired on at this stage by anger, or was it fear? I'm not sure. But I knew that if I did not refocus this energy it would turn in on me and destroy anything left that was good.

Barnes's words got me thinking about Chloë's life and what she had meant to me. And I thought a lot about time too. The illusion of time. I pondered Benjamin Franklin's words: 'A long life may not be good enough, but a good life is long enough.' For 15 years Chloë had lived a wonderful life. I wasn't fooling myself; that was not enough. But it was better than some children in the world. She got ill and that was really rubbish. But then she adapted and we skipped off again. I felt compelled to seal the years that we did have and to box them into something magical. They were far from wasted years and I have a treasure trove of fine memories that I can tend in my mind and take out when I need them. By giving myself permission to cherish the past, I opened a door to some kind of healing.

This thought was a real breakthrough moment for me. I could mourn what I didn't have; at the same time I didn't have to mentally destroy all the good that had happened. She had lived and I had been her mother. This helped me to bring some balance back into my life and started, what I believe, is the vital process of integrating the loss into the very heart of oneself. I knew the importance of this through my mother's early death. One day I looked in the mirror and saw my mother staring back. It was at that moment that I knew that all the goods bits of my relationship with her were still there. Only now they were deep within the essence of who I had become. I believe that this is critical to being able to survive/thrive after this kind of loss. I will never be anything but sad that my daughter died but I am starting to feel a new burning love for what I had rekindled inside of me and just sometimes this snuffs out the sadness. But not always and that's ok.

***

There is an analogy in yoga which I find helpful. One cannot get better at yoga by powering through or trying to be massively competitive. It doesn't work and it is a sure route to injury and more stiffness. The same with grief. I have found that one has to sit back and give into it. Don't try and fight it; just absorb the feelings and allow the sadness to drip through your veins. I found some peace when I accepted this. I became more aware of the general fragility of life and accepted that I was so floored because I had had something so wonderful.

Nowadays I find comfort sometimes. I can lay back and open my mind to memories of really good times. I can feel my daughter's hand in mine and listen to her chatting, laughing and yes I can almost talk to her. My husband too. Mostly I remember how funny he was, how he lit up the world. I read once that one doesn't stop having a relationship with somebody just because they've died. I've found this to be true.

The death of a child is like no other. A partner can, in the crudest sense be 'replaced,' a parent, by the natural order of things, fades into the past as the focus shifts to a new generation. A sibling is brutal. But having lost all of the above, nothing really compares with the loss of a child. Nothing.

I often think about the births of my two girls. Both were long labours. Hannah 26 hours. Chloë 24. My focus with Hannah has shifted more towards the young woman she is now as I have had the wondrous honour of watching her grow up. With Chloë I need those fine memories to carry on. The past has to be precious as it's all I have. I remember her birth like it was yesterday. How extraordinary the human body is. One moment I felt I was dying of exhaustion and then out she popped. Recalling that moment still sends a marvellous shiver down my spine. I had never felt more alive in my life. Never happier.

I held her to my chest and sobbed. I felt alone, but not lonely, and the luckiest person in the world. I fell in love at that moment. "I will keep you safe," I whispered as I gently brushed a curl from her perfect little face and she latched onto my breast. Just like Hannah we bonded immediately – how blessed was I. I thought back at all the stories I'd covered as a journalist of infant death, infant disability and glanced up to the heavens. I really thought it was going to be ok.

But it wasn't and I didn't keep her safe. And however irrational this may sound this is the thing that I'm still coming to terms with. I have felt a failure as a mother, even though I know intellectually that I didn't ever have the power to fight cancer in the first place. And is there some arrogance in me for ever assuming that I had any kind of control over the fate of my children's lives. But it's an uncomfortable pervasive feeling and I still struggle with it. I wonder if other bereaved parents feel the same?

***

Fast forward 15 years from Chloë's birth, I'm looking up incredulously at that sign, Teenage Cancer Ward. I'd visited these places as a reporter. Doing my job and then getting the hell out of there. These were places for other people, other families, not mine. I'm ashamed to say it never even crossed my mind. Families like mine didn't get cancer! Oh the arrogance, the naivety.

I can still sense that cloying smell, even now. A mixture of the toxic chemicals they pump into young veins. That mixed with disinfectant, fear and despair.

But let me not mislead you. I lost my child, so that place has dark memories for me. Nothing went right for us there. But with the benefit of the distance of time, I can now recall it as a wonderful place too. Full of the most extraordinary people who keep on going day after day, sometimes in circumstances that more resemble a war zone than a hospital. And one full of children and young people.

And as if that wasn't enough, they have to deal with parents like me. Angry, scared, desperate, needy. It would be fair to say that I was a real pain in the neck at times. But in my defence, I guess who wouldn't be.

***

As I've already said anger and despair seemed to be my primary emotions. I would quickly spin from one to the other. It felt like a kind of insanity. My anger just spurted out everywhere and hit many of the wrong people. I'm really sorry for that. For example, my bizarre fury at the work of the TCT; that it even existed. I hasten to add this was entirely illogical and I was completely wrong.

In reality the Teenage Cancer Trust does a fabulous job. It helps to bring joy into these young people's lives when everything has gone very dark. They get to mix with other kids in the same situation. Lots of celebrities visit. Something Chloë loved. Me, not so much. The cynical journalist in me felt some were there more for PR purposes than anything else. I think that was true for some, but definitely not for all. There are pool tables, arts and crafts, counselling and, most importantly, heaps and heaps of love and kindness.

One stand out moment, for me rather than for Chloë, was when Roger Daltrey, patron of the TCT, came into Chloë's room. By that time I absolutely refused any cameras in the room – no way was my daughter being the token child with a bald head in a publicity shot for a celebrity. Roger was completely unfazed and asked if he could come in anyhow. "Who is he?" whispered Chloë. "Can you sing *Pinball Wizard* for us?" I asked. "Sure," he said. And he did. Well, I'd always loved Roger Daltrey, but now he was my total hero. He had such presence, you could tell you were standing with someone special, but he was so normal and kind. "You've got quite a good voice," Chloë chirped as she glanced up. "Thank you very much," he said. What a guy!

But like everything there are difficulties too. Children die in this ward. It seemed to me at the time it was on a daily basis. More likely a monthly basis, in more measured hindsight. Imagine your own child. You are trying to keep everything as normal as possible, as light as possible and the absolute unthinkable happens – a child who has become your child's best friend dies. And then another one. And another. I will never forget Chloë's face as she suddenly realised she had an illness that other people, just like her, had and that they didn't always get better.

Another problem for me - and I know this sounds terrible but I want to be honest - was the children who did get better. And, to be fair, most children with cancer THANK GOD get better. But when your child is dying you feel excluded from this club too. Chloë always looked so beautiful and so well people never thought she was in the 'dying club' so parents would whisper to us about another: "That child is terminal." And there was some kind of survival mechanism that kicked in that pushed the other families away. As if the dying was going to be contagious.

This is a nightmare situation for the hospitals to deal with. They want to support the family of the dying child; but keep the spirits up of the rest of families. It is impossible to deal with all those deaths when you are down on resources whilst trying to care for your own child. I remember Bradley. A feisty young lad, full of bravado. Charismatic, cheeky. His dad was a prison officer. We got friendly. They were funny and we had some great evenings together. You get close in that ward. We all knew that Bradley was really poorly. He too had Ewing's sarcoma. It happened in a matter of months. One day he was telling us about all the escapades he'd been up to when not on chemo – this kind of language becomes everyday on this ward – the next he was lying dying in a bed. I couldn't bear it. I went to see him, against the nurse's advice. I knelt by his bed and held his hand. I'd left Chloë to do this. I remember the nurse's face. She was so shocked. She came over and very gently led me away. Looking me in the eyes she said, "No. You need all the strength you have for Chloë. We will look after Bradley."

She was so right and I wish I'd thanked her for that. It was one of the many every day thoughtful, kind gestures that I had got used to. With all its challenges our NHS is a wonderful thing. It makes me proud to be British. Gosh we must do everything possible to protect it. When your child is seriously ill you see it in its full splendour.

But. And I do have big but here. The main problem I had throughout my whole journey was a kind of 'us and them' mentality. I hated being called "Mum." I know minor, but it somehow stripped my personality away. I'd always gently correct, "I'm Debbie. Nice to meet you." I really think that this helped as suddenly somebody had to look at me as a person with a name.

Some of the battle weary doctors and nurses were not so easy to crack. They'd been on the frontline for years. They had to build up some kind of armour to protect themselves. Day after day looking into the eyes of desperate families as they had to say again and again, "Sorry we're out of options." It must harden people. And here lies a big difficulty. People are nowadays used to being treated like consumers. We like to be thought of as individuals with rights, preferences. Well at least I do. And if that doesn't happen we make a fuss.

If ever that behaviour is going to be switched on to full beam it will be when your child is ill. Generally we got the best care in the world and of course nothing is always going to go completely right. But here are a few things I want to list that almost brought me, already right up against the wire, to my knees. It was all to do with communication issues and not about funding. For some reason the funding issues e.g. there are very few pillows in NHS beds, didn't seem to faze me. And this wasn't just a question of me not having to worry about money. Us parents would often share pillows, fans, food; we all seemed to muck in and help out those who struggled more. It was rarely an issue

My list here is not a criticism but just an observation of how a parent under such stress can really be hurt by those little perceived injustices of life in an NHS hospital. I hope that these are somehow helpful:

- Hospital receptions. The first thing that us fragile families come up against. At UCLH there was a young man who ran the reception. No political correctness whatsoever. He'd bowl up to Chloë give her massive hug and ask when her next modelling assignment was. Chloë adored him and it always started our visit on the right footing. His warmth made the difference; it made us feel, 'Yep we can do this.' We felt we were human beings, not patients. Contrast that with another hospital receptionist who we saw every day for months and months. "Name? Date of birth? What are you here for?" Every day! She barely looked up. What I wanted to say was: "We're here for exactly the same reason as yesterday and guess what we have the same name!" What I did say, every day, is "I'm not prepared to discuss intimate details of my daughter's treatment here in a crowded reception." A couple of years later I met this woman again and she was absolutely charming. I doubt she ever realised how upsetting her attitude was at the time; especially to a super sensitive family. I think that is just a matter of better training isn't it?

- Then the Royal visit. William and Kate were opening a new ward for teenagers. In one of those nutty NHS decisions that seem so incredulous, my Chloë, a patient, was not allowed to visit the ward as it wasn't her day to have treatment. I guess nor were any of the other young people. Whoever was the visit for then! This time I swung into full action. I wrote to the Chief Executive and the Chairman. They were brilliant, responsive and I think furious on my behalf. I'm sure that this wasn't a deliberate policy of trying to exclude young people. It was just totally thoughtless. Chloë got her tickets at the front of the queue and she had a wonderful day with her sister Hannah chatting with William and Kate. It was a great day. But what about the children and teenagers who don't have annoying on-your-back parents? They are the ones that always seemed to get such a raw deal.

- The doctors who used words like, "We've been here before, we know what you're going through." They don't. We are all unique. How much better the doctors who said, "How does it feel?" or "How would you like to see this bit happen?" I have the most tremendous respect for people who qualify and work as doctors and nurses. But, it is important for both them and for us patients to be reminded often, that they are not Gods. They are doing an extraordinary job; but they are human beings with the same hopes, dreams and fragilities as the rest of us. Our journey worked best when a health care professional was confident and humble enough to admit to not knowing it all – they can't, the human body is too unpredictable. I was especially comfortable when a doctor just dealt with us as people and worked alongside us. And I'm quite certain this approach helps the doctor too; they don't have to take on all of the responsibility.

That said the goodness of the NHS seriously outweighed the bad. Our consultant Professor Jeremy Whelan - whilst we didn't always

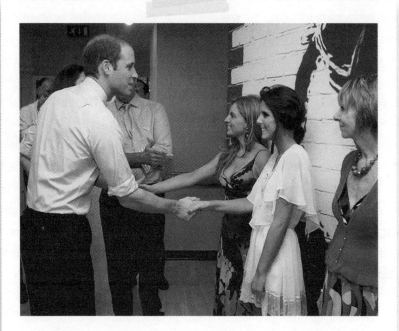

*Chloë next to Hannah, thrilled to meet William
and Kate at the Royal Marsden Hospital*

see eye to eye - was the best in the business. I have absolutely no idea how this man continues to work in this world, confronted day after day with hopeless cases and pleading parents. When he has to give up on a child, which he often must, he faces a parent like me. Furious, defeated, pummelled to the floor. He became, for a short while, the man I hated most in the world. At the time, second only to God. How could he have let my child die? Why didn't he try harder to make the medicine work?

In time I realised he was just a man, not the God that I had wanted him to be. He was at the mercy of a box of rusty old tools that were never going to make a difference. He, like my family and all the others, were at the mercy of a system that is well intended but doesn't bother to push down the barriers and ensure children get the best - not the worst - drug options possible. He was just at the frontline.

I gave him hell for a while. Including dragging him along to a meeting at the House of Lords with our local MP Paul Burstow. I felt he needed to explain himself. Why hadn't he saved my daughter? Looking back I was literally mad with grief. I would have blamed anybody who stood still long enough. And the kindly, expert, considerate Professor Whelan seemed to understand this. He turned up and took the punches.

He knows now that I am sorry about all of this. Anyhow this man was always way above an angry broken mother. He'd dedicated his life to caring for surely the most heart breaking cases imaginable. I am very glad that he was my daughter's consultant. I am sorry I was mean to him and now, as an extra apology, I raise money for his excellent charity.

*****

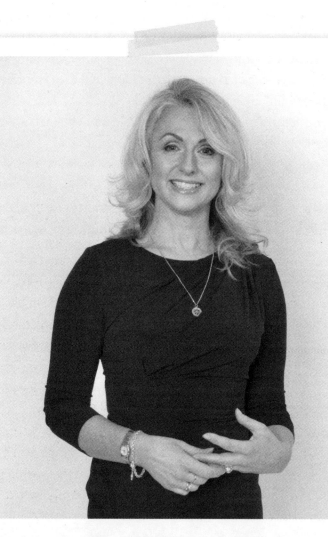

Since losing Chloë and then Simon, life has irrevocably changed but I've learned — am learning — to live a new life

'Courage is contagious. Every time we choose courage, we make everyone around us a little better and the world a little braver. '
 — Brene Brown, Texan researcher, storyteller

LIFE AFTER SO MUCH DEATH

MY daughter chose courage. At times she was terrified and so very sad at what she knew she would be missing. She had her life planned out. Drama and English at Edinburgh and then into journalism like her mum. She would dance and play her way through life. Sometimes she was angry, other times determined to live every second. It was her sadness that was so hard to cope with. She also, although she was rarely prone to being sentimental, knew how painful my life would be without her. I think children and young people really worry about this.

We never spoke about her dying. We both knew but we couldn't say it. It was beyond us. She once asked if the drugs didn't work could she be at home. A day before she died she suddenly remembered she hadn't taken the possibly life-saving pill. She could hardly swallow. "We'll miss today's dose."

***

I'm 55. Not young but not really old either. There is a unique feeling that arises after seeing a ward full of dying young people. Dying children. The horror and sadness is beyond words. How could somebody who has seen this not be grateful for having any life chances at all?

'Jump into the middle of things,
get your hands dirty,
fall flat on your face
and then reach for the stars.'

– Joan L. Curcio

I saw this in one of those little books about resilience and this jumped out too:

'When one door of happiness closes, another opens, but often we look so long at
the closed door that we do not see the one that has been opened for us.'
– Helen Keller

I guess when I think of my own gravestone I want it to capture something like this: "Despite everything I went out and gave it a shot." I admire courage and resilience in other people and I hope in my life I've demonstrated that I have some too. I would have hated to have lived a timid, little life. And I think I've fought a good fight.

So my darling daughter Hannah you have something to work with. I would like a little stone and to have my ashes buried with my daughter. I would like my words to inspire not to depress.

I have reached middle age. I had a wonky start. But since then, I've married, had children, had a fabulous career, great friends and I've been so loved. I have in some ways been incredibly lucky.

As I've said there were times after my daughter died that I longed for death. An end to the pain. But I don't anymore. Instead I feel I've reached a kind of peace with death. I'm happy to look it straight in the eye and say, "Oh yes I know you will come to me one day and I hope that I will be ready." I won't say, why me? That would be quite ridiculous for me. Through the death of my daughter I have discovered how to live well. To live with a kindness and compassion. To realise how true my Irish grandmother's words were "There's good in the worst of them and bad in the best of them."

***

Because of the tragic events in my life I believe I will now die well. At least I want to die well. Most importantly for the emotional health of the family I will leave behind. I could die a horrible death, with disability and uncontrolled pain. I know the reality of both of those things. But I hope that spiritually and emotionally I will embrace death in the same way that I have dealt with my healing from loss - full on honesty, connection and curiosity.

If I have cancer I want to book into the Royal Marsden Hospital in Sutton. The best of all hospitals. At least in my experience. I'm a passionate believer in specialist hospitals. We need fewer general hospitals and way more specialist ones - even if they aren't closer to home. I have worked extensively in the NHS as a communications consultant and know that we don't have this model because it doesn't work politically. It's too difficult a message to 'sell.' As soon as a government talks about changing models of care the easy message is 'save our hospital.' And this wins votes. A clear simple message. But it isn't simple. Some hospital A&E departments should close. Care isn't always best just because it's closer to home. Take a look at how stroke treatment has been transformed by specialist care.

Dear reader I beg you, if you have a serious illness get to a specialist hospital. They do things better.

So that's where I'd want to be. My plan would be to look at the evidence. Will this chemotherapy have any chance of working? If the odds aren't good I will not take it. Not at this age. I will look to palliative care and if necessary a hospice - the most wonderful of organisations (please give money to these as they are not properly government funded).

I'd take care at home too. I will fight you tooth and nail if you try and take me to a general hospital. These are places for people to get better, not to die. To die in hospital is cruel and shouldn't be happening.

I want my family to keep me in a beautiful room in my Clapham home. A home I love more than any other. I want fresh flowers around the bed and when times get harder I want to listen to the beautiful Hindu *Gayatri Mantra* or my favourite hymns *Silent Night* and *On Eagles Wings*. I will listen to Leonard Cohen, Bruce Springsteen and Nick Cave. I need the sun, the light on my face. I want to listen to the *Archers* and watch *EastEnders*. I want my family to read me poetry and Shakespeare.

I will say goodbye to my friends a good while before the end. There will be a handful of people around my bed. The people who have my heart. My daughter, my partner, my grandchildren and a few special friends. I know who they are and at some point I will write to them.

I have a lot of experience of death to draw upon. My mother's death was horrendous for me as a 20 year-old. It was shrouded in so much secrecy and fear. My big strong mammy had no skills to handle death and nothing to demonstrate how to do it. She was beaten and shrivelled into her death. She was utterly terrified and never openly acknowledged that she was going to die.

Times were so different then. Coming from a poor family in a different age childhood death had been a constant companion. As well as trying to rub off her Irishness, she had wanted to leave the death and darkness of the poor Irish background. A new start in England gave her the opportunity to paint a 'perfect world' for herself and her family. Her intentions were good but the pressure on us to live these perfect lives was so destructive. Life just aint like that.

When she died it was three weeks before my 21st birthday. I'd been bought up in a family with ludicrous expectations. I was a baby mentally and emotionally. I couldn't cook, I'd never been expected to do any cleaning whatsoever; I'd had no boundaries. The only rule was that I bought into the idea that our world was perfect and that wonderful things would happen. I think, I hope, I've painted a far more realistic, and therefore potentially much happier, picture for my own young.

My mother dying left me confused. To say the least. I didn't cry at her funeral, but I noticed my hand trembling. I hardly remember her funeral. My father cried and I just looked on bewildered. I had no idea what to do. My brother cried but turned to his friends for support. I didn't know where to go.

I have felt very alone in my life at times. But that moment was one of the worst. I didn't know anybody else who'd lost a parent and my friends, of which I had many, had no idea what to do either.

Aunties and uncles would disappear. I never knew where they'd gone and would often end up having nightmares about them popping up in my bedroom demanding to know how many Hail Marys I'd said before bedtime.

I had dreams of myself as a little girl alone in a huge field. I have a blue dress on that is way too big and the saddest face. I felt I had no defences, no structure, nothing to draw from.

But the beautiful thing is I knew how to love my own children so much. I started as a pretty dreadful mother, but realised early I needed to get my act together. They were too worthy of a useless, clueless mother. I knew I had to work hard to get it right. I read and read and read. I worked with therapists, doctors, nurses, to ensure that every step of the way I got better. And there's lots of work still to be done.

Hannah is currently reading the book *They F*** You Up: How To Survive Family Life* by Oliver James.

It's painful but it has opened up a refreshingly honest dialogue between us. I can explain why I did some of the things I did – like turning up late to pick her up from a school trip. I've not been allowed to forget that one. My life was too messy, I was doing too much. I slipped and it was entirely my fault. I need her to know how blameless she was and how life just somehow got in the way.

And I think in that I succeeded. With a hell of a lot of help I must add. Chloë did have a brilliant life whilst she was here and, if I dare whisper it, a good death. That is if death can ever be good for an 18 year-old girl. But my family, our friends, her friends, the doctors and nurses, the psychotherapists held her and we walked the journey with her. I never left her side unless she wanted me to. I went in with her to every scan, every MRI (the noise!) and it was the biggest honour a human being could ever have. I discovered the best version of me and that has really helped me deal with the horrendous aftermath of my daughter's death. Unlike with my mother there was never any denial, any running way, looking the other way, not being there for each other. For the first time ever in my life my family and I drew inwards around my daughter.

**

Now I truly understand the importance of truth and connection. And love. Isn't it all we ever have really?

There is one regret I have around my daughter's death. A lifelong people pleaser, I tried to consider others and let some people in who I didn't want there. They were nice people it's just it wasn't their place. And from this I would so strongly advise any fellow people pleasers to drop them NOW. This is your time, with your family. Be bold.

**

So back to my own death. As I move through my 50s, I so often hear of friends with horrible diagnosis. Seems so obvious really, the body gets older and rustier and finally breaks down. I hope I have many more years to live as I feel my experiences have been truly transformative and whilst I don't exactly spring though life with purposeful joy just yet, I'm working towards it. Through all the pain and heartache I have learnt how to live a good, purposeful life. And I've got back in touch with my compassion and kindness for other people. It's a wonderful feeling. I feel so much better placed to do something good in this world, to contribute. At the risk of sounding cheesy, to leave the world a tiny bit better than when I started.

***

My daughter Hannah is my biggest challenge. I know how much my death will hurt her and when I ponder my own death I can't help but think I will let her down again by dying. However illogical, I feel I let her down by not saving her little sister. My omnipotence didn't stretch that far I guess. Such arrogance really. My death will happen and I want to show her the best death possible - if I can. I would prefer not to have Alzheimer's or MND or a lingering long painful death. But I understand that this could happen.

And whatever does happen, I want us if possible, to plan collaboratively to part. To die in the best way possible, whilst ensuring that she stays as intact as possible. It is a personal belief but I do not believe my life is entirely mine to choose what to do with. I believe I have a duty to those I leave behind; to those who have honoured me with their love.

***

It could be that I opt for an assisted death. I've seen this up close and personal and it is nothing to fear. But I will ensure that I would only do this with my family's blessing and I know the pain and the unresolved feelings that can be left after this choice.

Choosing an assisted death is not for the faint hearted. To actively take hold of one's fate takes giant balls! But to live in the face of chronic disability, illness, decrepitude, well isn't that brave too? My objection to my late husband's death is that it was not collaborative and it did not feel gentle or graceful. It was so much less about us as a loving couple and more about an audience. I think that my husband needed this as the intimacy of a death would have been too painful for him. I loved and admired my husband greatly. He was not a cruel man and was hugely dignified. But - and I seek only to show a truthful picture - his death felt very much like abandonment and that it wasn't a collaborative act.

I'm afraid I don't care if any of this sounds selfish. Aren't we all a bit selfish? It is the truth of my situation and all I can do as a writer is bring you my truth and hope is some way it may help somebody somewhere at some time.

Assisted death is not suicide, but it feels a hell of a lot like it to me. And I know that you may well say, "Well so what."

***

THE DEATH TOUR

I recently went on what I lovingly call The Death Tour. I spoke at a local Catholic school about assisted dying. The young people were 17. It was an inner city state school and was, I'm proud to admit, a 'tough gig.'

My fear that the students would be bored by these old codgers going on about death was instantly dismissed. We showed Simon's hour and a half documentary. The room was entirely silent. Apart from a growing sound of muffled sobs.

These feisty, brilliant, energetic young people were gripped. I made the case against assisted dying. Friend Simon, who was brought up an orthodox Jew and now describes himself as an atheist, spoke in favour.

Another friend David, a lawyer and a judge who lost his only son Daniel to the same cancer as Chloë, spoke of the importance of hope in end of life care.

These kids stunned me in so many ways. Their engagement and raw honesty. Gosh don't we underestimate young people sometimes. They were asked to vote before the talk and then again afterwards on whether they were for or against assisted dying. The head teacher predicted "us Catholics do a pretty good job of indoctrinating our kids" and guessed that the vote would be about 70 per cent against and 30 per cent for before the talk, shifting to about 60 per cent for and 40 per cent against. We all nodded in agreement.

Wrong. The students voted overwhelmingly in favour of assisted dying (85 per cent) before and voted almost the same way at the end. But crucially at the end they expanded on their thoughts with comments like, "I think it would be ok for others, but not for my mum" or, "I think it's ok, but not in England." I took this as a victory as I think the simple case for assisted dying is actually a way more powerful one. But to me it is its simplicity that is the problem. Humans are messy, life is messy and when things come to it they tend to be a hell of a lot more complicated than we think.

Asked a simple question the students came up with a simple reply. But pushed to delve beneath the surface and put themselves into somebody else's shoes, the views were far more nuanced and thoughtful.

***

So that's where I'd want to be. Through all my campaigning work on childhood cancer and through my many journeys through so many different care pathways I know that whilst modern medicine can perform miracles, there is so much it cannot do and so much it still cannot cure. Ultimately in my experience the challenge with illness has been emotional and spiritual. How does somebody try and live the best life possible in a shrinking more challenging landscape. I am glad I have got to reflect so deeply on this issue. I'm bemused when I look back at the old me. The one who thought that my family were above any kind of illness. The one who thought that life would go on forever and that career, status and money were important. I have become more humble, more thoughtful and as a by-product of it all, happier and richer – in an emotional sense.

I was having a medical test a few months ago. It was a screening but an important screening for somebody with my family background of cancer. I trotted in in my smart work suit. I was terrified; I needed all the emotional armour I could muster. Glasses on. Briefcase. Whilst I claim no fear of dying, I am left with a pathological terror of hospital tests. It's the one thing I can't reason myself out of. It brings back all the memories. The moment we stepped over the line with Chloë. With Simon. The line from ordinary life into the gloom of being a patient. I know it will come for me at some point but it won't be easy. There are too many memories… Not yet, I whisper. Please. I now have more to do.

The doctor was very pleasant and chatted through everything. He spoke to me like a fellow professional; little did he know that I felt about an inch high inside. "I'm utterly terrified,' I finally admitted. "Really?" he looked puzzled. "You look so calm and it's only a screening test. At this point." And then I told him. I had that feeling he would understand. I told him my story. A hardened consultant, or so I thought, he fell back into his chair and clasped his hand over his mouth. "I'm so sorry. I just would never have known looking at you." When I had the procedure he'd put in big letters at the top of the page "Nervous patient. Maximum dose of sedation." I was delighted. Everything was fine and he treated me with a new warmth. I revealed my vulnerability, he responded and it all felt ok.

***

I know my story is extreme. And I am quite sure that there will be many people who just don't want to read it. But I think/hope that there are others who will. Who may be stuck in the pit of some kind of human despair; there are so many different types. I hope that they will come on my journey with me and end it thinking, "Well she's got through and there's some light. Maybe I can too." For as this book has been so cathartic for me, when I think of what I hope it will really do, it is this. Simply put I hope it will help somebody else feel that there is always a way through however awful things get.

At night I often read *If* by Rudyard Kipling, one of my favourite poems. It has been recently heavily criticised but I still love the simple sentiments within it.

'If you can meet with Triumph and Disaster
And treat those two impostors just the same...'

***

So dear reader here I am. When it all started I never thought I'd ever get to this place. My heart is still in tatters, how could it not be, but it is now part of who I am. I feel like a patchwork quilt made up of a multitude of terrible and wonderful memories. The result is that I have finally sewn some kind of life, some kind of persona together. I look in the mirror and I am now proud. I see a strong woman who has survived. Not a perfect one by any means but one that I like. Now that is a good feeling.

*****

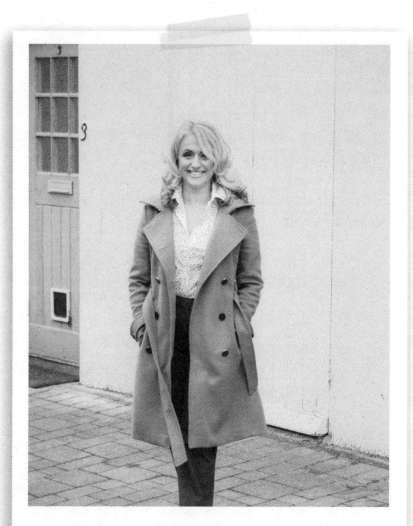

Me, today

'We must be willing to get rid of the life we've planned, so as to have the life that is waiting for us. The old skin has to be shed before the new one can come.'
—Joseph Campbell

THE NEXT CHAPTER

WRITING my story has been so cathartic. It has allowed me to place the good and bad in little boxes in my mind. It has helped me to separate and to remember that life has been breathtakingly marvellous as well as heartbreakingly horrible. This has been key to my survival; finding some kind of balance in the narrative of my life.

I wanted to write this book from the moment that Chloë got ill. I wanted to chart the journey, as I thought that this could be really important for others. Then Simon happened and it got left on a shelf for a while longer.

Now it is complete, I feel ready for the next chapter of my life. Writing has helped me to structure the pain and to place it within the boundaries in my mind. Early on I realised I wanted to ensure that I could remember Chloë, and then Simon, in a way that demonstrated what they had meant to me; but at the same time mindful that the force of the pain could destroy everything good in the landscape ahead of me.

Until Chloë got ill I'd had a great career but I hadn't always felt that I had a clear view of where I was going. I felt I kind of lurched from one thing to another and often thought that the dream job, dream life was just over there, just out of reach. Through Chloë's illness and death I had to change; I had to shift the way I saw things. I had to think really deeply about myself, what worth I had in the world and how I spent every single minute. In honour of my beautiful, courageous daughter I needed to ensure that my legacy would be worth it. That I was somehow worthy of her and all that she had borne and suffered.

My book is the first step. My first achievement in this brave new world. I hope it helps other people, as this has been the intention, alongside allowing me to make some sense of what has happened. However sad my story is I think - I hope - it's uplifting too. I have survived and on some days I even thrive. How about that? I am a better person and I have a rock solid focus on where I want to go next. I work from good intentions, get things spectacularly wrong sometimes and try to not get knocked off my perch so often. I care deeply what my friends and family think of me but I have really little time for people who want to squash me down or veer me off path. In short I don't mind if people don't like what I have to say or do. I will now only ever do what I think is right. I hope that I am a walking, talking example that us human beings may not be able to control what happens, but we can control our given attitude in any circumstances.

***

Writing has also taken me in a completely different direction and it's pretty exciting. I spent a lot of time reading and researching evidence and views on resilience and well-being. I have been especially interested in how other people have managed after catastrophic events. This has led me to further study and I'm about to embark on a Master's Degree in Applied Positive Psychology.

Oh and I've found love again. It happened one day and happened so surprisingly easily. I was certainly not expecting that. I've moved house and am building a new life and a new home. My old friends have a very special place in my heart and always will. But I find myself making new deep friendships again. This amazes me, how many wonderful people there are out there. Some of my best evenings are now with a group of women at my local tapas bar. We drink sherry, laugh and enjoy the moment. I now know how precious these moments are.

And Chloë and Simon. Well they stay so close. I talk about them every day, I think about them every minute. It has become very much part of who I am. The most feared question for us bereaved parents, "How many children do you have?" Easy now. "I have two children. Two girls." And if I choose to, and if I want to, I will tell them all about my daughter Chloë. But only if they are special enough.

*****

MY READING LIST

LITERATURE has saved my life on more than one occasion. That feeling of anticipation, excitement as you open that first page and start a whole new relationship with your author. Here are some of the books that have given me comfort and allowed me to find insight and meaning at the worst of times.

ON ILLNESS, GRIEF AND LOSS

History of a Suicide - Jill Bialosky

When Things Fall Apart - Pema Chodron

The Year of Magical Thinking - Joan Didion

On Smaller Dogs and Larger Life Questions - Kate Figes

On Death and Dying - Elisabeth Kübler-Ross

On Grief and Grieving - Elisabeth Kübler-Ross and David Kessler

When Bad Things Happen to Good People - Harold S Kushner

A Grief Observed - C.S. Lewis

In a Dark Wood - Joseph Luzzi

With the End in Mind - Kathryn Mannix

A Manual for Heartache - Cathy Rentzenbrink

Sad Book - Michael Rosen

Grief Works - Julia Samuel

***

TO FIND MEANING AND COMFORT IN THE WORLD

Levels of Life - Julian Barnes
Man's Search for Meaning - Viktore E Frankl
Ammonites and Leaping Fish: A Life in Time – Penelope Lively
Gilead - Marilynne Robinson (anything by Marilynne Robinson)
The Beginner's Goodbye - Anne Tyler

***

USEFUL ORGANISATIONS

aPODD - www.apoddfoundation.org - a wonderful charity which focuses on finding cures for as many childhood cancers as possible.

Child Bereavement UK - www.childbereavementuk.org – a fantastic organisation and my charity of choice. Child Bereavement UK supports families and educates professionals when a baby or child of any age dies or is dying, or when a child is facing bereavement.

Little Princess Trust - www.littleprincesses.org.uk – provides natural hair wigs for children suffering hair loss from illness or treatment.
The Teenage Cancer Trust - www.teenagecancertrust.org

*****

ACKNOWLEDGEMENTS

THERE are so many people to thank in bringing this book into being. I had totally underestimated the task of pulling something like this together and the huge amount of help and support I would need from my nearest and dearest.

Most importantly I want to thank my dear friend and publisher Shoba Ware, the founder of Splendid Publications. I first met Shoba at the start of our careers when we were enthusiastic young reporters on the Croydon Comet newspaper. She has remained a dear friend ever since. But she's also a consummate professional and a hard task master when it matters. I was given no special treatment due to the length and depth of our friendship and she has guided me with a stern, but tender, hand; encouraging when I needed it and with the occasional push when I lost focus. There is no way that I would have been able to produce this book without Shoba by my side; somebody I trust entirely and respect so much. An outstanding friend, woman and publisher!

***

Thanks to the families I lived alongside for quite some time. The families who have or have had children with cancer. I've stayed in contact with some and the others I've never forgotten. Your bravery changed me forever. I'm now lucky enough to work alongside other parents across Europe and beyond as we never stop campaigning for better treatment for children and teenagers with cancer.

***

I can never truly convey my gratitude to the people who worked in the NHS. The doctors who worked around the clock to make sure that we got a chance of some kind of life. The doctors and nurses at University College Hospital, The Royal Marsden Hospital in Sutton, Croydon University Hospital. A special mention for the nurses from Croydon's Hospital at Home team. They stood out for me as beacons of compassion, kindness and professionalism.

***

In Simon's journey I thank Doctor Erika Preisig. A noble woman indeed and one who lives life by her rules. Respect.

I'm not sure that I've seen a better medical team in action than the team from the MND clinic at King's College Hospital. Dr Rachel Burman you are the best.

***

Special mention to my friends for being so supportive and encouraging of my project. For all your words, and acts of kindness, over many years.

***

ACKNOWLEDGEMENTS

But mostly thank you to my amazing daughter Hannah and those two little people Roman and Nahla. To Sarah, Chloe's dearest friend, who will always be a central figure in our close knit family. My biggest supporters and my best friends. And last, but by no means least, to Tim, my new partner who has sat patiently by whilst I've spent so many evenings, holidays and middle of the nights glued to my computer. We're now on a whole new journey together and it feels so hopeful.

*****

Also available from Splendid Publications

How to Survive Divorce
By Anthea Turner

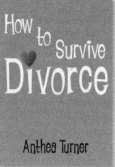

TV presenter Anthea Turner was devastated when her husband Grant Bovey cheated on her with a woman young enough to be his daughter. Although both she and Grant had left their previous partners for each other, Anthea was convinced they had both learned from their mistakes and were destined to grow old together. Heartbroken, she filed for divorce.

How to Survive Divorce is Anthea's candid take on the emotional toll the end of her marriage took on her well-being and how she eventually came out of the ordeal, a stronger, more confident woman. Open and honest, she pulls no punches as she describes falling apart in the months after the split and turning to her friends, family and professionals to help her through her darkest days.

This is a book which has been carefully researched and written by the star and is full of helpful tips and real-life case studies. How to Survive Divorce aims to offer women who find themselves facing divorce – whether or not from choice – practical help and guidance in navigating what can be a legal and emotional minefield. From choosing the right solicitor to getting back in the dating game, this is a must-have guide on how to survive divorce and come out the other side.

£9.99 (paperback)

Daniel, My Son -
A Father's Powerful Account Of His Son's Cancer Journey
By David Thomas

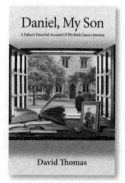

Daniel was just 17, rich of talent and full of dreams, when he received the devastating news that he had bone cancer all over his body. In pain and facing horrific treatment, his chances were slim. But Daniel refused to give up on life and studied Classics at Oxford, played with the BBC Symphony Orchestra, line-judged at Wimbledon and was chosen to carry the Olympic Torch.
Meanwhile his heartbroken parents scoured the world for a cure and learnt to navigate the medical maze. Their mission was to create hope – for Daniel, themselves and all those facing the same nightmare: a child with cancer. This is a father's powerful story of his love for his son and humankind's overriding need for hope.

£7.99 (paperback)